RADIOLOGY MANAGEMENT

A GUIDE FOR ADMINISTRATORS, SUPERVISORS, AND STUDENTS

VOLUME 1

Eric Bouchard

SHEPHERD ᴉɴᴄ

10340 MILITARY RD · P.O. BOX 1861
DUBUQUE · IOWA · 52004-1861

BOOK TEAM

Pat Swanson Eichhorst *Project Editor*
Angela M. Timmerman *Interior Layout*
Doug Flint *Cover Concept and Design*

SHEPHERD ᴵⁿᶜ

Judith A. Shepherd *Chief Executive Officer*
Stephen E. Shepherd *President/Publisher*
Marie L. Schmitz *Vice President of Operations*
Terri L. Schiesl *Production Manager*
Martin J. Lange *Director of Marketing*

ISBN Volume 1 1-881795-04-7
      Volume 2 1-881795-05-5
      Set   1-881795-06-3

Manufactured in the United States of America.

10 9 8 7 6 5 4 3 2 1

*This book is lovingly dedicated
to my daughters, Erin and Lauren.*

CONTENTS

VOLUME II

SECTION THREE PLANNING   1

SECTION FOUR MANAGING   117

Preface

In 1983, my first book titled *Radiology Management: An Introduction* was published. It was my belief that students and new radiology managers wanted a straightforward, practically-oriented text to use as a guide to the daily operations of a radiology department. The book had a wide appeal to instructors, students, and practicing managers. Nearly nine years later, I met radiology managers who said they were still using that book!

Obviously, the point had been reached where further development and refinement of the useful information found in the first book was necessary. The dynamic changes in radiology management over the last decade required that alteration, deletion, and expansion of previously-presented material be made.

The result was a new book, *Radiology Manager's Handbook*. When it was in final preparation in the spring of 1992, Mary Jess of Shepherd, Inc. called to say...."You need to find a stopping place, this book won't fit in a one inch binding!" So I stopped sending material to the publisher but I didn't stop writing and collecting my radiology management "pearls."

In this second edition, the string of pearls gets longer with over 50 separate new illustrations and chapter sections or appendices. Don't think of this updated version, *Radiology Management: A Guide for Administrators, Supervisors, and Students Vol. 1 and 2* as strictly new editions but as additions to my attempt to bring a concise yet comprehensive desk reference to the busy radiology manager.

The purpose of this handbook is to introduce the reader to a subject area and offer useful examples easily adapted for use in today's radiology department.

It is my hope that this handbook will stimulate further interest in radiology management as a field of study. I believe that radiology management is a dynamic and changing field and that this text offers practical, useful applications in the "real world" of radiology management.

Eric Bouchard
July 1993

Acknowledgments

Thanks to Michael Stephen Kuber again for his permission to reprint "Radiology Administration: Structure and Style." Thanks to Mary Louise Wright for her permission to reprint information on radiology reimbursement and to Sandra Harrison for her help with career ladders. The American College of Radiology has been very gracious in allowing me to use material on contract media management, reporting and mammography. Rick Martinez of *Administrative Radiology Magazine* allowed many uses and citations, and Peter J. Bartolazzi contributed valuable information on equipment specifications. Credit also goes to Jim Dohms of Sarasota, Florida for the chapter he contributed on hazardous materials, the RMBA for coding and nomenclature for stereotactic breast biopsy, *Second Source Imaging Magazine* for an extensive figure describing the current state of bone densitometry and the department of nursing at Baptist Hospital of East Tennessee for assistance with the career ladder discussion.

Blaine Lester of Johnstown, Pennsylvania contributed two figures for employee selection, and the directory of technologist education in MRI originally appeared in *RT Image Magazine*. Alan Weinstein contributed the new chapter on Radiology Benchmarking and Monica Langley of Knoxville, Tennessee helped with ADA as it relates to hiring. I am also grateful to Anthony G. Lyon, M.D., for his encouragement, and I am deeply appreciative of the numerous sources of adapted material in this text. Finally, I need to mention that the inspiration for this project comes from my long time association with the American Healthcare Radiology Administrators.

Special thanks to Pat Eichhorst at Shepherd for expert editing, careful proofreading and attention to all those last minute details.

Eric Bouchard, FAHRA

About the Author

Eric Bouchard, B.S., M.A., R.T. (R) is the Director-Center for NeuroSciences and Rehabilitation at Baptist Hospital of East Tennessee, Knoxville, Tennessee. He is also a Fellow of the American Healthcare Radiology Administrators and has previously published both books and articles on the subject of radiology management.

INTRODUCTION

This book on the subject of radiology management is a compilation of information on topics relevant to anyone interested in radiology management. The book is organized under four major sections with subheadings listing subjects often unique to the field of radiology management. As the field of radiology management has grown sophisticated, so have the information needs of radiology managers and students. Today's busy radiology departments have leadership at numerous supervisory levels. These levels of expertise have a knowledge of radiology management that is varied. What is particularly attractive about a handbook-style treatment of this subject is quick reference. Instructors also find this format useful since each section can stand alone and information can be gleaned from selected areas. In particular, practical lessons and examples that the radiology manager may adapt are prominent aspects of this handbook.

The content of this book is a straightforward treatment of subjects specific and unique to radiology management. No attempt is made to present a topic in its entirety; rather, radiology managers will find the concise approach to various subjects a very attractive feature of the book. As much as possible, subjects included in this handbook are on the cutting edge of radiology management.

The material is organized under the administrative functions of people, technology, planning, and management. The length of each of the 46 sections varies depending upon the difficulty of the subject. The book contains charts, graphs, and examples. A major characteristic of this handbook is the use of descriptive materials.

The most distinguishing feature of this book is the way in which the material is organized. This is the only handbook-style treatment of the subject of radiology management published today. This quick reference-style text will benefit the reader because of the ease with which information about a specific subject can be found. This book is an indispensable reference for managers at all levels and students too.

The author

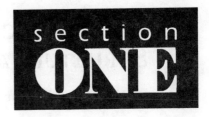

PEOPLE

1.1 RADIOLOGIC ADMINISTRATION: STRUCTURE AND STYLE

Contributed by Michael S. Kuber*

Birth of a Profession

Professional Radiologic Administration has risen from the ranks of an informal apprenticeship to a highly specialized radiologic management science. Being scientifically oriented, radiology managers are continually acquiring the most modern techniques and skills to effectively manage the radiologic enterprise.

In the past we have been a very individualized entity. Aside from significant technological changes, radiologic activities and practices have come under external forces which have exerted influence and demanded change from the traditional ways of radiologic management. The very nature of these influences has challenged our professional practices. As a result we now find ourselves confronted with economic, social, and governmental pressures and regulations.

In view of such forces, a greater internal force has developed within our own ranks for competent, qualified, and formally trained administrators to manage radiologic activities.

Historically, certain management theories and practices have been established as foundations for management practices. With these basic foundations and through advanced preparation, education, and experience, managerial talent can develop an effective management style to meet the needs and demands of the radiological enterprises.

As the industrial revolution has proceeded on its course and technology has changed the face of the entire medical business world, one thing has become clear: There is a great deal the modern

*This article on basic management functions originally appeared in the Winter 1980 issue of *Radiology Management*. It is reprinted here with the permission of the author and publisher. After a decade of reviewing the literature of radiology management it remains a fine example of general management principles applied to the specific requirements of radiology administration.

medical business world can do without. One thing it cannot do without is an adequate number of skilled and effective administrators.

Managerial talent to manage increasingly complex departments and technology is becoming a more scarce and critical commodity. In large part, this scarcity derives from an inevitable increase in the level of skill and expertise demanded of an effective radiology manager, but it is no less a scarcity. The basic level of drive, experience, and systematic advanced preparation (usually through formal education already accepted as indices of potential for selection of a manager) is constantly being raised. Upgrading of managerial qualifications is being forced at every level of the radiology operation. Even those administrators appointed to positions designed to test, develop, and season them for future assignments must now be a higher quality of entrant. It is no longer feasible to rely on trial and error as the principal method for developing future administrators. Administrative resources are increasingly more scarce. The selection and development processes themselves must be managed.

The key to success in allocating scarce administrative resources is in developing useful measures and indicators which will tell when a need exists. An important strength of developing such measures and indicators is that it suggests a variety of objective measures which may be used at a number of levels for screening administrators. The particular advantage of measures and indicators of such a nature is that they are relatively objective in quality. With the aid of developed indicators, through observation, and through investigation of performance, one should be able to identify specific administrative styles.

Over a period of time, through education and experience one can build a foundation for a personal, effective administrative style. Such criteria for a foundation may be a blend of the following factors: the range of time in which plans are made, the reliability with which deadlines are met depending upon whether they are long-term or short-term, specificity/objectivity versus generality/breadth of personal and business goals of subordinates, methods used to analyze problems, decision-making style and theory, extent to which the administrator's manner is cool and calculated versus emotional and spontaneous, professional affiliations, and personal belief in business and economics.

It is difficult to understand the perspective of the radiology manager without considering the manner in which he is selected, educated, and initiated into the world of medical healthcare administration. In early American radiology, administrators received their training largely through apprenticeships or on-the-job experience. Such exposure included little formal teaching. Related administrative responsibilities were those delegated from the appointed chairman-administrator, who rarely was questioned in his administrative style or practice. This practice of management was continually supported in the past by the traditional view that matters of radiological concern are to be decided upon solely by the radiologic chairman.

With the rapid growth and advancement of radiology, there developed certain social, cultural, economic, and governmental influences that confronted and challenged the traditional view of radiologic management. Due to these influences, physician-administrators were confronted with challenges of a magnitude that they had never before experienced. (Almost every area of radiologic activity—in ethics of practice, distribution of services, allocations of cost, assessment of quality, recruitment into the field—has now come under scrutiny and re-evaluation.) Although physician-administrators possess medical and technical expertise and competence for practice in their field, they no longer can hold a monopoly on wisdom in matters concerning the department's organization, distribution, and economic nature.

Such changes have summoned many of the administrative procedures and practices to consumer review. Now, more than ever before, physician-administrators are agreeingly bowing aside and setting the stage for professional radiologic administrators.

With the advent of the professional radiology manager comes a new and potentially exciting career that demands expertise, education, field experience, and the talent to develop in oneself an effective managerial style. The following discussion, therefore, concerns itself with just that domain.

The field of study termed management is concerned with the process by which resources including machines, money, materials, technology, and people are coordinated to achieve predetermined goals. The recorded literature which comprises the field of radiology management includes many different viewpoints of the most fruitful manner in which to study and approach management. Each viewpoint proposes a particular definition which emphasizes one or more aspects of management. For example, one viewpoint places emphasis on the process of achieving goals through the efforts of people. Another emphasizes management as only one aspect of group behavior, while a third describes the technical aspects of coordinating and focuses on the elements of coordination as the function of management. Other definitions and viewpoints can and have been drawn, but the essential point of recognition is that the field of radiology administration is far from settled.

The unsettled nature of the field reflects not only the complexity of administration, but also the relative newness of scholarly interest in radiology administration. The complexity of the management process requires a great deal of knowledge and understanding. Administrative management is a fundamental human activity which defies easy analysis. In fact there now exists no one general theory of administrative management which serves to consolidate and direct efforts of researchers and practitioners. However, certain accepted basic characteristics have been long established through time, education, and experience. Existing theories as well as newly formulated administrative management theories often fail to describe the key issues of "what" administrators actually do.

Aside from management being a distinct kind of activity or process, it can also be spoken of in terms of a group or class of people. In these terms, one's immediate thought is that of attributes and qualifications of that group of people who rise to be administrators. Some of the most common traits displayed by these people are such qualities as: a history of personal betterment and a high level of energy, drive, motivation, and insightfulness; being able to deal with problems and preside over change; a zest for living; and a rich foundation of experience backed by formal, related education. These characteristics of an administrator or his patterns or beliefs, attitudes, and values set the tone for his department in all of its relationships with hospital administrators, employees, patients, suppliers, and the public at large.

Functions of Management

Another way of understanding administrative management styles is to examine the functions of management. The administrative process comprises the functions of: 1) planning, 2) organizing, 3) staffing, 4) leading, and 5) controlling.

1. **Planning** is the ability to effectively look ahead to the future, set goals, determine policy and procedures, and establish the methodology of accomplishing these goals. The cognitive and decision-making processes are heavily involved in planning.

2. **Organizing** requires the departmental breakdown of total work to be done into jobs, groups, and department specialties, and the establishment of workable relationships between these areas. It includes such things as the use of technical staff, setting up of jobs, establishing patterns of communication, and determining authority and responsibility relationships.

3. **Staffing** refers to recruiting and selecting the appropriate experienced technical and support staff to man the radiology department.

4. **Leading** is the motivation and direction of people to achieve departmental goals and objectives.

5. Finally, the **controlling** function includes measurements of work performed, comparison of performance with predetermined goals, objectives and standards, and initiating corrective action when necessary to ensure that performance meets standards.

In analyzing the skills needed by radiology managers, it is fair to speak of three types which seem to reveal and re-enforce themselves in a recently-conducted radiological managerial inquiry of selected mideastern radiology hospital facilities. These three attributes are technical, human, and conceptual skills. Technical skills refer to proficiency in handling methods, processes, and techniques of a particular department or departmental unit. Human skills are those which provide the ability to work effectively with others and build cooperative group relations to achieve departmental goals and objectives. Conceptual skills denote the ability to perceive the department as a whole and to recognize interrelationships among its functions and to be able and capable of effectively guiding the department in consideration of the multitude of forces affecting it. Such skills are concerned with the realm of ideas and creativeness.

During such development of conceptual skills and administrative styles, it is most important to keep in mind that human beings, as individuals, are very complex in their psychological nature. While there is still much to be learned about the nature of man, what is known and understood should be incorporated to complement an administrative style.

Planning

The primary function of administrative management is **planning** and the technique of planning. This objective includes all managerial activities and efforts which determine results and the appropriate means to achieve results. We might call this managerial function "advanced thinking as the basis for doing." There is a variety of themes reported in administrative literature which attempts to classify the stages of the planning function. These can be condensed into the following four phases of planning. Phase one entails establishing departmental goals and classification of these goals by priority. Phase two requires the administrator to forecast future events which may affect accomplishing goals. Phase three materializes phase one and phase two, as well as aids in making the plans operational through budgeting. Phase four communicates and implements policies which direct activities toward required goals.

The initial step in planning is the determination of goals. In doing so, administrators are concerned with three aspects of goals: priority, timing, and structure. It is readily accepted that the priority of goals implies that at a given point in time the achievement of one goal is relatively more important than others. Since the resources of any department must be allocated by rational means, it becomes quite clear why the establishment of priorities is essential. The other aspect mentioned is that element of time which implies that the department's activities are guided by different objectives dependent upon the duration of the action. The traditional framework for these time spans are: short-term, intermediate, and long-term. These describe periods covering one year or less, one to five years, and five years and beyond, respectively.

The structure of goals is the dynamic process of breaking down the department's activities into units, for example, by modality specialties. In this structural division, each unit is responsible for attaining its goals and objectives, whether they are reflected in terms of workload or patient care.

It then becomes readily apparent that as an administrative practitioner develops and initiates his departmental goals and objectives, he must integrate those needs to reflect the needs and desires of his personnel. A committed administrator possesses not only a desire for a successful organization, but also a responsibility for helping his personnel enjoy a more meaningful work life. Through conceptual skills, he acknowledges that today's employee has matured in an era of affluence, secondary schooling, and college education. In addition, the employee expects more and has more to contribute to his work life. Today's employee is less submissive and seeks more influence over affairs in his place of employment.

With such knowledge in mind, the skillful administrator creates an alignment of goals and interest between his department and its manpower force. This requires a pervasive process of developing and refining departmental goals. Goals that are specific objectives are defined and established for the department and its individual manpower force. These goals and objectives can evolve through departmental staff meetings, where such goals (and goal activities) can be structured around the employee and the department. Authority is delegated down to many levels, giving the employee a real sense of responsibility and control over his life within the department.

Such an approach invokes a sense of responsibility and control, inducing the worker to a real personal commitment to those goals and objectives. This administrative approach holds that people will exercise self-direction and self-control in working for objectives to which they are committed. They will become committed to working for the departmental goals to the extent that they gain real satisfaction from doing so. The implications are clear: Team building and participative management are essential factors to the contemporary administrator.

Forecasting, the second phase of the planning process, is a critical step in the implementation of goals. The results of forecasting are included in budgets which are major planning documents of a department. Two basic issues are of concern during the forecasting phase: 1) the expected level of departmental activity during the planning stages and 2) what levels of resources will be available to support the projected departmental activity.

The third phase of the planning function is budgeting for resources, revenues, and expenditures. Such budgets account for personnel, equipment, maintenance, and supplies. As well as serving as a planning technique, budgets are also used as a controlling device.

The principal means by which administrators implement plans is through policy-making, the fourth phase of planning. Policies, like plans, are both specific and general, abstract and concrete, short-term and long-term. Policies are statements which reflect the basic objectives of the department and provide the guidelines for carrying out action throughout the department. The ultimate test of a policy's effectiveness is whether it leads to the intended objectives and goals.

The planning function then refers to administrative activities that determine, in advance, goals and the means for achieving them. In a practical sense, the determination of means for achievement of goals involves the assignment of tasks to people who must then complete their work in a coordinated manner.

Organizing

The administrative process of the **organizing** function achieves a coordinated effort through the design and structure of task and authority relationships. The two key concepts of this function are design and structure. Design refers to the conscious effort an administrator makes to predetermine the way in which work is to be executed by his staff. Structure denotes relatively stable relationships and aspects of the department. Thus, we can describe this function in terms of dividing tasks, departmentalizing tasks, and the delegation of authority over such tasks.

The organizing function can easily be depicted by development of a departmental flowchart which delineates design and structure. When research evidence is examined, it appears that there exists a variety of organizational approaches to structure and design. However, the evidence itself does not allow conclusive statements to be made concerning which type of design is best suited for a particular department. It does indicate, however, the type of administrative and nonadministrative personnel, the type of work being performed, the size and work activities of the department, communication flow patterns, as well as other essential features. Such features or variables should be given more than just passing attention in the design of the radiology team unit.

Controlling

The third distinct function comprising the administrative process is that of **controlling**. Controlling incorporates all activities which administrators undertake in attempting to assure that actual operations conform to planned objectives and goals. The desired effect of administrative control is a stable work force which pursues its prescribed or planned activities with a spirit of initiative and sense of unity. The means to those ends would then include staffing the department with a competent administrator and an experienced and qualified technical staff, augmented by the use of rewards and sanctions. It therefore appears that implementation of control requires three basic conditions: 1) standards must be established, 2) information which indicates deviation between actual and standard results must be available, and 3) action to be taken to bring about correction of any deviation from goals and objectives.

The control function then involves the implementation of methods which provide answers to three basic questions: What are the planned and expected results? By what means can the actual results be compared to the planned results? What corrective action is appropriate from which authorized person?

Preliminary control focuses on the problem of preventing deviations in the quality of departmental resources. Concurrent control monitors actual ongoing operations to assure that objectives are being pursued. Its principal means of implementation are directing or supervising activities. Feedback control focuses on end results. This type of control derives its name from the fact that historical results guide future actions. Thus, the controlling function consists of the development of techniques which bring about planned-for results, and the overriding administrative responsibility is to integrate these three functions into a coherent management process which enables the department to achieve the levels of performance expected by the elements of the medical society that sustain it.

Leading

To this point we have discussed the **planning, organizing,** and **controlling** functions of a radiologic administrative practitioner. But in order for any department to be successful and thrive effectively, **leadership** is essential. Whether or not a leader is effective depends on the results achieved through his practice of leadership. The success of leadership is measured by the performance of the leader's unit. An effective administrative leader can influence followers so that they achieve the highest level of performance possible with the skills, resources, and technology available. Leadership is a complex process associated with numerous theories and models. Leadership thus can be described as the process of influencing others to act to accomplish specified objectives and goals. In other words, leadership is an attempt by a person to affect or influence the behavior of followers in a given environment.

Effective leaders move subordinates to action by a number of methods: persuasion, influence, power, threat of force, and appeal to legitimate right. Leading involves a close personal relationship. Face-to-face interaction is a major ingredient of leadership. This implies that a person in a leadership position must transmit his feelings and exhortations to his subordinates by the process of communication. Communication involves sending, receiving, and understanding messages. The way in which subordinates respond to a leader's initiation of actions will affect his manner of leading, as well as his effectiveness. Leadership literature defines leadership influence in terms of power, the control which a person possesses and can exercise, or the ability to obtain dominance of objectives and measures. Now, a review of the five most widely accepted bases of power is in order. These power bases are as follows: coercive power, reward power, legitimate power, expertise power, and referent power.

Coercive power is based on fear and the expectations of individuals that punishment is the consequence for not agreeing with the actions, attitudes, or directives of an administrator. It goes without saying that an effective and successful administrator has no need for such a power base in his administrative style. Reward power is the subordinate's perception that compliance with the objectives and goals of his supervisor will lead to positive rewards. Utilization of this power is seen through recognition of a performance well done. Legitimate power stems from the position of a superior in the departmental hierarchy and is analogous to authority. Expertise power is that power based on some special skill or knowledge. This power base is usually limited to a specialized area of activity—that of the expert's specialty (for example, administration, angiography, or ultrasound). Referent power has as its basis the ability of subordinates to identify with a leader and may be influenced by such factors as emotion, admiration, etc.

Recognizing that there is no one single most effective leadership style for generating good performance from the departmental unit in all situations, one can reasonably ask, "What style works best in what setting and situation?" The perceptive administrator may be able to diagnose accurately the demands of the situation and alter his behavior somewhat to meet the varying situations. Alternatively, it might be possible to restructure the work environment so that a leader who feels comfortable practicing a particular leadership style can be most effective in a situation suited to him. In any event, some of the more prominent situational dimensions in determining leadership effectiveness are as follows: 1) leadership style, 2) followers' expectations, 3) task structure, and 4) power position of the leader. These dimensions imply that the administrator holds a clear view and understanding of his department and of his employees' perspectives.

Staffing

Finally, and most importantly, is the foundation and backbone of any department—its staffing. **Staffing** or manpower planning is the process by which a department ensures that it has the right number of people who possess the properly-related skills at the right time to perform jobs and technical procedures useful to the department and the population that it serves. This is accomplished by the development of a concept of the department as a structure or system. In view of the long-term scarcity of high-caliber talent in the labor market, especially of technical, professional, and managerial personnel, the function of manpower planning takes on considerable importance.

Principal activities involved in manpower planning are as follows: audit the present labor force in terms of skill mix, experience, and location; create a viable method for forecasting manpower needs giving consideration to present volume of departmental work, anticipated departmental expansion, and changing technology; decide critical skills and establish plans for their allocation; analyze the labor market and trends in supply/demand relationships; and develop programs for meeting manpower shortages. Since the human resources of any radiological department are its most important assets, it goes without saying that the caliber of the work force largely determines the department's strength and its success as a medical enterprise.

Conclusion

Administrative practitioners of radiologic management recognize that the simple question, "What do managers do?" often elicits simple answers, such as, "They manage." Radiologic administrative managers are integral aspects of the radiology enterprise, yet often their roles are taken for granted.

The aim of this presentation is to provide the reader with a concept of management style and structure. The author has chosen to develop the concept of management style and structure because of the fact that a concept is usually an abstract idea or meaning based on a particular set of instances. As such, a concept is apt to change depending on who shares certain ideas, under certain situations. A fundamental aspect of management is that its meaning has changed and will continue to change over time. To suggest anything else would imply a definition or relatively fixed idea, which is simply not the case. Instead, a discussion of management theory and its principles, such as **planning, organizing, controlling, leadership,** and **staffing,** are reviewed in hopes that readers will incorporate such principles as a basis for developing their own concept and style of effective radiologic administration.

1.2 THE MANPOWER SHORTAGE IN RADIOLOGIC TECHNOLOGIES

Ask any radiology manager if a shortage of qualified radiologic personnel exists and the answer will be an emphatic, yes! Recent surveys by the American Hospital Association and the American Healthcare Radiology Managers suggest that the answer to that question is overwhelmingly affirmative. The shortage is national in scope and is illustrated by vacancy rates up to 15 percent for radiographers, 13 percent for nuclear medicine, 17 percent for sonographers, and 21 percent for radiation therapy. Hospital radiology managers certify these numbers with 91 percent of these managers reporting vacancy rates across the board in their departments.

Current staffing levels indicate a need to train more radiation workers, yet training opportunities in the United States are on the decline as well as the enrollments in these schools. What factors are causing this difficulty in attracting new people to careers in the radiologic technologies? The shortage is a result of fewer people entering the field, combined with a growing demand for more radiation workers brought about by an aging population. In addition, managers report that job burnout among currently employed technologists is increasing attrition from the profession. Clearly, the answer to this supply and demand question is to increase the number of persons entering the radiologic technologies. According to the Summit on Manpower, a Washington, D.C. based coalition of 19 national healthcare organizations, 6,000 technologists are needed per year when currently only 4,000 to 5,000 are being added to the market. The Summit, which has validated the widespread perception that a shortage exists, has concluded that existing data on manpower in the radiologic technologies indicate that the supply of qualified personnel does not meet current needs and will not meet future needs.

Defining the Field

"Radiologic technologist" is an umbrella term for a variety of jobs that involve examining patients with medical imaging. Training typically begins as a radiographer, a generalist who performs x-ray examinations. Radiographers may further specialize with additional training into other areas such as nuclear medicine, medical sonography, or radiation therapy technology. Other specialization areas include work in computed tomography, magnetic resonance imaging, and special procedures. The Summit uses the following discipline descriptions from its 1989 task force on data.

Radiography

The radiographer is primarily responsible for applying ionizing radiation to demonstrate portions of the human body on a radiograph, fluoroscopic screen or other imaging modalities to assist the physician in the diagnosis of disease and injury.

Nuclear Medicine Technology

The nuclear medicine technologist uses radioactive materials in specialized studies of body organs and/or laboratory analysis to assist the physician in the diagnosis of disease and injury.

Radiation Therapy Technology

The radiation therapy technologist uses ionizing radiation producing equipment to administer therapeutic doses of radiation as prescribed by the physician for the treatment of disease.

Sonography

The sonographer may provide patient services in a variety of medical settings in which the physician is responsible for the use and interpretation of ultrasound procedures. In assisting physicians in gathering sonographic data, the diagnostic medical sonographer is able to obtain, review and integrate pertinent patient history and supporting clinical data to facilitate optimum diagnostic results; perform appropriate procedures and record anatomical pathological and/or physiological data for interpretation by a physician; record and process sonographic data and other pertinent observations made during the procedure for presentation to the interpreting physician; exercise discretion and judgement in the performance of sonographic services; provide patient education related to medical ultrasound; and promote principles of good health.*

*Summit on Manpower: Report April, 1989.

Reasons Behind the Shortage

The reasons for the current manpower shortage among radiation workers must be understood if realistic strategies are to be developed to effectively alleviate the impact on the quality and safety of radiological healthcare. The reasons for current and anticipated shortages include but are not limited to the following:

- Lack of public knowledge/awareness of the radiologic professions.
- Impact of the PPS reimbursement system has resulted in hospital cost cutting, hiring freezes and decreased lengths of stay.
- Changing demographics: a decline in the 18 to 25 age group leading to decreased enrollment in allied health educational programs.
- Disinterest in healthcare careers as many other job opportunities now exist that attract women (nearly 80 percent of the healthcare work force).
- Increased educational requirements for entry level positions.
- Increased requirements for licensure or certification.
- Alternative employment settings other than hospitals.
- Concern about work hazards, radiation, AIDS, malpractice.
- Lack of opportunities for upward mobility.
- The expanding elderly population and its special needs.
- Better pay for professions with similar education requirements.
- Changes in personal priorities of individuals for more leisure time and regular working hours (a nine to five schedule).

What a Manager Can Do About the Problems

It is the responsibility of the manager to communicate to hospital administration the seriousness of the manpower situation and to take a proactive stance in promoting strategies to relieve these shortages for the future. Some ways to help find solutions to the shortage are described here; the key is participation and personal commitment of time and energy to this critical professional issue.

- Participate in a comprehensive, collaborative state-wide strategy to address health manpower issues with your hospital association.

- Establish a fixed authority to convene the persons necessary to deal with solutions.
- Identify and publish scholarship opportunities for training in the radiologic technologies.
- Create more opportunities to reach elementary, junior and high school students with information on radiologic careers.
- Analyze current recruitment and retention methods in your own workplace.
- Develop more creative retention strategies (i.e., job analysis, paid education leave, tuition reimbursement, child care, flexible benefits, job sharing, career mobility, eliminate salary "compression" and implement career ladders).
- Focus recruitment effort for better students in less traditional applicant pools—minorities, older students, career changers and men.
- Encourage more practitioners to enter the work force through liberalization of licensing requirements and reciprocity.
- Reinforce current efforts to attract technologists by forming recruitment committees and establishing strong monetary incentive programs.
- Encourage the use of technologist extenders to perform the duties not requiring professional expertise.
- Develop opportunities for volunteers to expand their roles beyond those traditionally observed.

1.3 JOB DESCRIPTIONS

Good managers make the most efficient use of the human talent that they have available. A good job description allows the accurate and objective measure of an employee's performance. Evaluation of job performance takes place when a comparison of actual behavior is made to written standards contained in the job description. The success of a performance appraisal depends on the job description; without it the manager has no way to determine how well the job has been done and no valid way to issue raises or promotions. In addition, the purpose of the job description is to gauge the significance of the position compared to all others in the organization. The job description determines the part of the organization's objectives that will be accomplished in that position, defines why the job exists, and describes what accomplishments will be rewarded.

The Job Description and the Individual

When an individual is hired, a number of related factors should be defined, such as the duties and responsibilities of the job, the relationships with other employees, and the philosophies of the organization. A network of job classifications describing the roles of people within an organization provides an abstract view of the workplace. However, the organization is intangible; no work can be done until people are employed to fill various roles. The job description, an analysis of the specific tasks that give the organization structure, is one of the basic components of a healthy, functioning organization.

Prospective employees need a clear understanding of their obligations to the employer. Job descriptions should be available to applicants before they make the decision to accept a position. Written job descriptions assist recruits in interpreting positions. The results of their interpretations have a great influence on their job performance.

One important reason for an up-to-date job description is its value in directing and defining employee duties. The job description is also useful in forming a basis for discussion between applicants and the employer that will help applicants decide whether the job suits their personal requirements and abilities. Another useful function of up-to-date job descriptions is their use in settling disputes regarding labor relations. Labor problems, when they occur, stem from elements of the three main aspects of a job being out of congruence. (See Figure 1.1)

These three basic aspects are reward (wage and benefits), an opportunity to form relationships with coworkers, and an obligation to perform satisfactorily.

These three aspects of the job are the areas on which the average employee will focus. The third aspect, that of obligation, embodies the purpose of the job description. The employee is informed of the responsibilities of the job and understands the standards of performance. For the manager, arranging for rewards and promoting good interpersonal relationships among employees are important mana-

Figure 1.1   Job Congruence

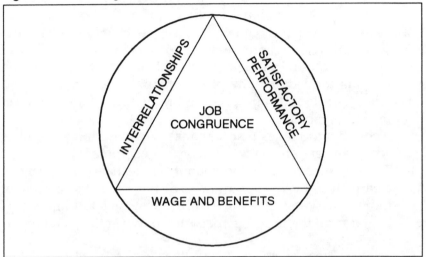

gerial responsibilities. The manager must emphasize to the employee the importance of accepting the obligation to perform satisfactorily.

The job description, in its most elementary form, is a list of the required duties and responsibilities for a particular position in the organization. An effective job description has four basic subdivisions: heading, job summary, duties performed, and general qualification requirements. The job description should be a realistic representation of the job functions. Some hints for writing effective job descriptions are suggested by the following principles:

1. Arrange the duties in a logical order. When describing a definite work cycle, such as a radiographic examination, the duties should be listed in sequential order. When the work involves a variety of related tasks, they should be listed in descending order of importance.

2. State separate duties clearly and precisely. It is inappropriate to go into detail about any of the duties described in the job description. If this were done, the job description would be very cumbersome.

3. Begin each sentence in the duties-performed position of the job description with an active verb. Examples of such statements

might be: "Load the automatic film changer," or "Adjust the radiographic control panel with the proper technical factors."
4. Be as descriptive and quantitative as necessary. Remember to state duties clearly and avoid ambiguous statements. Instead of "perform routine radiographic examinations," write "position patients for radiography of specific points of anatomy and select the safe and appropriate technical factors for exposure of the radiographs."
5. Avoid brand names that may make the description obsolete when changes are made in the type of equipment used.
6. Try to be specific about the amount of time that will be spent on a particular activity. For instance, do not say that 50 percent of the radiology assistant's time will be spent transporting patients to and from the radiology department when that is all that is required.
7. The use of the word "may" should be limited. It will confuse the employee when the job description states the employee may perform a duty, but is seldom, if ever, asked to perform it. Use of the word, however, can be a saving grace in any job description when the closing statement in the duties-performed section states that "the employee may be required to perform other duties as designated by the supervisor."

Job Title

The job title is selected to distinguish the job from all other positions in the department. It should be a title that is acceptable to the employee, because a title is closely tied to an individual's self-esteem. Selecting the appropriate job title is an important factor in motivating employees. The employee's role perception in the department, and the status and recognition that is received, can be directly related to the job title.

The title will describe the principle demands made on the individual in the position. The title will distinguish the position from all others in the organization and suggest that work assignments for the position are measurably different from all other jobs.

An excellent source of job titles is the *Dictionary of Occupational Titles and Job Descriptions.* This publication may be obtained through the United States Department of Labor. It can also be found in most college libraries. Another excellent source of job titles specific to diagnostic imaging is available from a publication entitled *A Position Description Development Guide for Diagnostic Imaging*. This guide may be purchased from the American Healthcare Radiology Managers.

Job Summary

The job summary is a brief one paragraph statement of what the job entails. The job summary will communicate the central purpose of the job. Like the job title, it will show how the job is different from all others. For example:

Staff Radiographer—Job Summary
The staff radiographer performs radiographic examinations of selected portions of the anatomy as requested by the clinician. The radiographer is expected to perform a variety of procedures with the knowledge and ability to apply a prescribed amount of x-radiation for the purpose of obtaining diagnostic-quality radiographs.

Duties Performed

The body of the job description lists the duties of the job in a logical order. It often specifies the way in which the work is to be performed. The duties-performed section specifies the required activities of the job. The reader of the job description may interpret the duties-performed section as examples of the work. The duties-performed section of the job description should be "criteria based." They will be based upon objective standards of performance.

General Qualification Requirements

The general qualification requirements of the job should include a list of the minimum acceptable standards. The list of personal qualities and experiences generally include level of education, work experiences, and evidence of personal initiative and ingenuity.

The ADA and Job Descriptions*

The Americans with Disabilities Act, one of the most sweeping employment laws in the last decade, is changing the way employers structure jobs and hire new workers.

The ADA protects current and prospective employees from discrimination based on their mental and physical disabilities. Disability-based discrimination is prohibited in virtually all aspects of employment—hiring, firing, promotion, pay, training, etc.

The ADA is unique among anti-discrimination laws because it can require employers to take affirmative action and incur additional costs in order to provide employment to employees with disabilities.

It is not enough simply to treat an individual with impairments the same as non-disabled persons.

Because of the breadth of ADA's coverage of private-sector employers, Congress delayed its effective date after passing the law in 1990.

The Equal Employment Opportunity Commission, the agency charged with enforcing the law, has indicated that protected disabilities may include orthopedic, visual, speech or hearing impairments; epilepsy; cancer; heart disease and diabetes. Also covered are mental ratardation, emotional illness, specific learning disabilities, HIV infection and drug addiction (although persons currently taking illegal drugs aren't covered).

The ADA protects an individual with disabilities "who, with or without reasonable accommodation, can perform the essential functions of the employment position that such individual holds or desires."

There are several steps in determining whether an individual with a disability is qualified for a position.

The first step is a determination of whether the individual meets the basic qualifications for the particular position. The employer can set necessary skill, experience, education and other job-related requirements of a specific job.

For example, an employer can legitimately require a secretary to type at 60 words per minute, so long as the business actually requires this standard for all secretaries. Also, the standard can't be established for the purpose of excluding those with impairments.

The second step in deciding qualification is to determine if the employee or job applicant can perform the "essential functions" of the job.

A written job description, which was used when advertising a job opening, may be used as evidence of the essential job functions. The employer's judgment as to which functions are essential will also be considered, as well as the consequences of not requiring an employee to perform certain functions.

Another factor to determine if a function is essential is amount of time spent. For instance, if an employee spends a majority of time at a cash register, this would be evidence that operating a register is an essential job function. On the other hand, although not much time is spent on the function, a firefighter not being able to carry out an adult from a burning building has serious enough consequences to mandate that this function be essential nevertheless.

The next step is determining whether an individual with disabilities can perform the essential job functions with a "reasonable accommodation" by the employer.

Such an accommodation is any change in the workplace or in procedures to permit a worker with disabilities to enjoy equal employment opportunities. If an employee or job applicant can perform the essential job function with certain reasonable accommodations, the employer must provide the accommodations unless they would pose an undue hardship on the business operation.

Reasonable accommodations required of employers can vary greatly depending on the job and impairment involved. They may include making existing facilities readily accessible to persons with disabilities, restructuring jobs or implementing modified work schedules, or buying special equipment. An example might be providing a telephone set with an amplifier for someone with hearing impairment.

However, the ADA doesn't require employers to make accommodations that would be unduly costly, extensive, substantial or disruptive. Also, accommodations for disabled aren't required if they would fundamentally change the nature of the business operation.

---

*From Langley, M. ADA Expected to change jobs, hiring. The Knoxville News Sentinel. June 27, 1993.

More About Criteria-Based Performance Standards

All healthcare organizations are striving to become more efficient; competitive pressures of the market and current reimbursement methods have placed new emphasis on appraising employees' performance. In many organizations greater than 50 percent of the operations budget is spent on employee compensation. Consequently, there is a move towards performance appraisal systems that will better assess performance. Unless the job description accurately reflects the major functions of the job, an appraisal cannot provide pertinent feedback. Criteria-based job descriptions offer the following advantages:

- Objective observable standards of performance.
- Prioritized job expectations.
- Allows managers and employees to target specific work behaviors.
- Ties performance to pay in an objective manner.
- Provides performance standards that will aid in:
  —interviewing applicants
  —orienting new employees
  —cross training
  —job delineation
  —counseling and discipline.

In order to move toward an objective approach to job descriptions, a set of performance standards for each job in the department must be written. A performance standard is a statement of the end result expected from the carrying out of a specific part of the job. A standard of performance is not a statement of the job duty. For example, for a radiology messenger a job duty may be: *Delivers radiology reports daily.*

A standard takes the job duty a step further by specifying an expectation for performance, such as: *Accurately delivers radiology reports to nursing units by 11:00 a.m. daily.*

The duty has been converted into a standard by specifying two expectations: *where* the report is delivered, and *when* it will be delivered.

Types of Standards

Most standards can be categorized into one of four areas; namely, quality, quantity, time, and process. Jobs that are task oriented are easier for which to write standards; other jobs where both technical skills and interpersonal relations are required may need some creativity to formulate into measurable standards.

For ease of understanding, the four areas of performance standards are defined here:

- Quality: a statement of *how well* a duty is performed.
- Quantity: a statement of *how much* work is performed.
- Time: a statement of *when* a task is performed.
- Process: the expectations as to *special steps* or *procedures* necessary to complete the job.

Elements of a good performance standard include stating an *end result* from the employee such as: "Performs routine radiological examinations so as to minimize the occurrence of repeat exposure." The second element of a good performance standard is that it be *specific*. The third element is that the standard be *observable*. Traits such as attitude, initiative, and flexibility are notoriously subjective. They may be made observable, however, by specifying specific behaviors. For instance, attitude may be quantified by applying a written standard that measures courtesy by monitoring the incidence of valid patient complaints (e.g., one or two in a six-month period. The fourth element of a good performance standard is *attainability*; to be compared against an unattainable standard is demoralizing to the employee. The last element of a good performance standard is *employee acceptance*. Obtain employee input to the standards before the standards are in place and operational. In summary, there are five elements that determine a good standard of performance:

- It states an end result.
- It describes specific activities.
- It is observable.
- It sets a reasonable expectation that it is attainable.
- It is understood and accepted.

Writing standards of performance is the art of specifying supervisory expectations and assigning relative importance to these expectations. The key to success in writing valid performance standards is involving employees in the process of formulating those standards. Achieving "buy in" with positive discussions about what the job entails will lead to the best set of performance standards for your work environment.

The employee is the best source of information about the job and how it is performed. A manager can be guilty of writing an idealized job description. The employee has first-hand knowledge of what the job actually entails. Providing the employee with a form for updating the job description is the most effective method of collecting the necessary information. A sample form is illustrated in figure 1.2.

Figure 1.2 A Survey Form Useful for Updating Job Descriptions

---

**JOB DESCRIPTION REVIEW
SURVEY FORM**

1) EMPLOYEE NAME: _____

2) JOB TITLE: _____

3) DEPARTMENT: _____

4) SUPERVISOR: _____

5) Describe the general responsibilities of your job. Please summarize your job in 100 words or less.

6) State specific duties that you perform daily. Try to list duties you frequently perform first. It is also helpful to list your duties according to decreasing importance. Use extra sheets of paper if needed.

7) Do you operate any special equipment? If so, list equipment and its frequency of use.

8) How much supervision do you receive? Does your supervisor review your work hourly, daily, weekly?

9) Do you supervise any personnel? If yes, how many and what are their job titles?

10) What do you consider to be the necessary qualifications for your job? That is, what is the minimum degree of preparedness an individual must have to be successful in the job?

Elements of Job Enrichment

Job enrichment requires that the manager take responsibility for re-evaluating jobs to ensure that the employee remains involved in meaningful activity.

A well-conceived job provides an arena for self-fulfillment for the employee, while it assures increased productivity for the employer.

Job enrichment incorporates change that moves in a positive direction for the employee. Changes redesign content and responsibility within a job. Content changes that lend variety and challenge to a position are vertical. "Vertical loading" allows the employee to assume more responsibility and requires a greater depth of understanding. Increased responsibility in a job allows employees to make decisions about how the work should be done. The employee then becomes accountable for performance and the resulting productivity.

Job enrichment provides opportunities for individuals to achieve growth through challenge and increased responsibility. Concerted endeavors to apply job enrichment programs in radiology departments will help boost the professional status of radiographers. When planning job enrichment, dimensions that need to be explored are: the employee's tolerance of responsibility; the employee's attitude toward working in groups; the level of complexity with which the employee can work; drives for security; and the employee's preference for supervisory authority.

Goals of Job Enrichment

The results of job enrichment are role enhancement and an environment that stimulates growth, self-actualization, and motivation. Some basic principles to keep in mind regarding job enrichment are the following:

1. Stimulate the employee's desire to learn and to advance by designing a job that is interesting and enables growth as the interests of the employee expand.

2. To personalize the job, make maximum use of the employee's skills. Also provide new skill-development opportunities; incorporate new skills in job content.
3. Give the employee control over the immediate job environment. Set realistic goals and deadlines.

Management's Responsibility for the Valid Job Description

If for no other reason than to comply with the law, a valid and reliable system of job description review should be in place in your organization. For example, valid job specifications are linked to the following legislation:

- Equal Pay Act (1963). For work to be considered similar, the jobs must be proved to involve equal skill, equal effort, equal responsibility, and be performed under similar circumstances in the same workplace.
- Fair Labor Standards Act (1938) involves the administration of overtime pay for after 40 hours per week. Job descriptions clarify which category exempt (salaried) or nonexempt (hourly) employees are placed.
- Civil Rights Act (1964). A well-described job and the requirements for that job are the defense against unfair discrimination charges.

To summarize, in addition to legal compliance requirements, management uses the job description for recruitment, selection, performance evaluation, training, compensation, safety and career planning. These functions cover the major areas of concern for human resources management. The job description as a management tool is possibly the most important piece of paper in the organization. This management tool will assist management to:

- Objectively show employees where they stand.
- Provide recognition for good performance.
- Improve communication.
- Clarify job objectives and performance standards.
- Identify training needs.

- Set goals for employee development.
- Identify unsatisfactory employees.
- Identify employees who show potential for promotion.
- Tie pay to performance.

Appendix A—Job Descriptions

Position Title—Radiographer

Job Summary

The radiographer performs radiographic examinations of selected portions of the anatomy as requested by the referring physician. The radiographer provides radiologic care to patients for the purpose of obtaining diagnostic quality radiographs for interpretation by the radiologist.

Duties Performed

Job Duty	Relative Weight %	Performance is good when:
1.	30%	Performs radiographic procedures in accordance with department protocols and procedures within standard time frames.
2.	30%	Maintains equipment in good operating condition and operates equipment according to department and manufacturer's recommendations.
3.	10%	Prepares and orients patients to the procedures they will have.
4.	20%	Is cooperative and helpful in a clear and courteous manner to coworkers, staff, patients, and visitors.
5.	10%	Maintains and exhibits a current knowledge of radiologic technology and participates in professional continuing education.

General Qualification Requirements

1. Graduate of an AMA approved school of radiologic technology.
2. Current registration and licensure (where applicable).

APPENDIX B

Position Questionnaire

Data for Job Evaluation Process

Name of Employee _____ Date _____

Department _____ Immediate Supervisor _____

Current Position Title _____

Purpose of Questionnaire

This questionnaire is designed to assist in describing the duties and responsibilities of positions. It will provide current and complete information on the incumbent's position and serve as the basis for equity in the job evaluation process. (To be completed by employee and approved by supervisor.)

A. Purpose of Position
State briefly the principal purpose or goals of the position—what it is designed to achieve.

_____

_____

_____

_____

_____

_____

_____

B. Basic Duties and Responsibilities
   In the spaces below, please list normal duties and responsibilities
   for this position. Describe each task, including *what is done*, and
   how it is done, and the *percent of total hours* devoted to each task. (The
   total of all percentages should equal 100%.)

Duties and Responsibilities   **Percent of Time**

1. _____

   _____

2. _____

   _____

3. _____

   _____

4. _____

   _____

5. _____

   _____

6. _____

   _____

7. _____

   _____

8. _____

   _____

C. Knowledge, Training, and Special Skills Required for Assignments in this Position. Indicate what is required and why it is necessary for successful performance of duties and responsibilities.

_____

_____

_____

_____

_____

D. Working Relationships
List the individuals (and titles), department, organizations with which you have the most frequent business contact. This should include contacts both inside and outside the hospital. Briefly describe the nature of these contacts.

Most Frequent Contact   Nature or Purpose of Contact

1. _____   1. _____

   _____   _____

2. _____   2. _____

   _____   _____

3. _____   3. _____

   _____   _____

4. _____   4. _____

   _____   _____

5. _____   5. _____

   _____   _____

E. Other Supporting Information
Please indicate any additional information you think would be helpful in understanding the nature, scope or purpose of this position.

1. Equipment and Materials
What are you required to use or operate in your position and for what purpose?

_____

_____

_____

2. Work Leadership/Guidance Direction
Do other positions/employees depend on this position for work assignments, training, advice, or guidance? Indicate the nature and frequency of such activities.

_____

_____

_____

3. Additional Comments

_____

_____

_____

This information has been completed and reviewed as follows:

Employee Signature _____ Date _____

Supervisor's Signature _____ Date _____

F. Environmental Requirements/Conditions—Accommodation of Disabled Workers (to be completed by Supervisor and attached to each employee's Position Questionnaire as appropriate)

1. Location

   _____

   _____

2. Access to Work Site

   _____

   _____

3. Climatic/Atmospheric Conditions at Worksite

   _____

   _____

4. Manual Requirements (Lifting, Climbing, Standing, etc.; Indicate Frequency)

   _____

   _____

5. Noise/Vibrations

   _____

   _____

6. Other

   _____

   _____

   _____   _____
   Supervisor's Signature   Date

Appendix C

Essential Job Functions			
Position: Radiologic Technologist/Diagnostic Section			
List the functions of each job in the columns. Answer yes or no for each question, making comments when necessary.			
Questions	**Function:** Produces high quality radiographic images	**Function:** Provides explanation to patients regarding procedure being performed	**Function:** Assists patients on/off x-ray table	**Function:** Continue in this manner until all functions have been listed
Must this function be done?				
Can other employees do it if the incumbent cannot?				
Would taking away this function fundamentally change the job?				
Does the job exist to do this function?				
Is special training or education required to perform this function?				
Is registration/licensure required to perform this function?				
Would there be any significant consequences if this function is not done?				
Do persons doing similar work in other hospitals perform this function?				
Time per week (in hours) to do this function.				

From: Wedel, C.S. The Americans with Disabilities Act: The Impact on Radiologic Technologists and Managers. *Radiology Management*. 15(2):23, 1993.

Appendix D

Six Steps to Accommodating Disabled Employees*

1. Analyze the particular job involved and determine its purpose and essential functions.
2. Consult with the individual with a disability to ascertain the precise job-related limitations imposed by the individual's disability and how those limitations could be overcome with a reasonable accommodation.
3. In consultation with the individual to be accommodated, identify potential accommodations and assess the effectiveness each would have in enabling the individual to perform the essential functions of the position.
4. Consider the preference of the individual to be accommodated and select and implement the accommodation that is most appropriate for both the employee and the employer.
5. Consider the ramification on the morale of peers and staff in general as a landmark ruling by the manager or director of the department.
6. Guarantee an environment free of recrimination, retaliation, prejudice, coercion or retribution with respect to the disabled employee.

1.4 SELECTING PERSONNEL

The selection of personnel is a critical operational responsibility for managers. The process of effectively selecting personnel requires that certain information be collected and be understood by the person seeking a new employee. The skills, abilities, and aptitudes necessary for a candidate to be successful in a job should be determined.

The selection of new employees depends upon organizational needs and must comply with legal hiring practices. Discriminatory practices in recruiting, testing, and offering of a job are illegal as defined by the Civil Rights Act of 1964 and the Equal Opportunity Act of 1972.

---

* Source: Equal Employment Opportunity Commission, "EEOC Title I Regulations and Interpretative Appendix," p. B-43. From Aribisala, EB Applying the Americans with Disabilities Act to Radiology. *Radiology Management* 15(2):27, 1993.

The selection of personnel is a procedure that culminates with securing a successful employee from an applicant pool. The procedure is also designed to eliminate unqualified candidates early in the process. The actual selection process is a series of steps. It starts with initial screening and ends with the orientation of the new employee. Figure 1.3 illustrates these steps in the process.

Job Analysis

At the heart of any organization is the set of jobs performed by its employees. All jobs need to cohere, to coordinate, and to apply directly to the mission of the organization. Job analysis involves the formal study of jobs. There are three basic steps in the analysis of a job:

1. Distinguishing the job from all others in the organization.
2. Identifying the duties and responsibilities of the job.
3. Assessing the requirements for successful performance in the job.

A job analysis results in a job description and specifications that serve as a guide for selecting applicants against measurable criteria. Job analysis provides answers to questions such as:

- How long does it take to perform the tasks that comprise the job?
- Why are certain tasks grouped together and how do they become the work to be performed?
- Is there opportunity for job redesign that will enhance employee performance?
- What are the behavioral characteristics of successful employees performing this job?
- What are the skills, traits, and experience required for candidates best suited for the job?

Figure 1.3 Selection Process

Preliminary Screening
Completed Application
Interview
Testing
Reference Checks
Employment Decision
Job Offer
Orientation

The use of job analysis is comprehensive and is an essential feature of the human resource function in any organization. Of particular importance, job analysis is specifically linked to legislation such as the Equal Pay Act (1963), Fair Labor Standards Act (1938), and the Civil Rights Act (1964).

In addition to legal compliance requirements, job analysis is deeply rooted in human resource programs and in activities as described by the following personnel functions:

1. **Job Descriptions**—The job analysis process updates and refines descriptions already in place.
2. **Job Specifications**—Individual traits and characteristics needed to perform the job are revised.
3. **Recruitment**—is useful when searching for the best candidate to fill a position.
4. **Selection**—Job duties and responsibilities are clearly outlined and matched to applicant's skills.
5. **Evaluation**—The analysis suggests acceptable levels of performance for a job.
6. **Training**—is conducted to satisfy the competencies required in the job.
7. **Compensation**—used to compare and compensate jobs.
8. **Safety**—establishes safe procedures in order to perform the work.
9. **Job Design**—used to structure and modify the job as organizational requirements change.

Finding the Qualified Applicant

The preliminary interview in the employment office of your organization sometimes precedes the completion of the formal employment application. When the selection process occurs in this order, an explanation about the application helps the applicant to avoid misconceptions about the information desired. The screening procedure involves informing applicants of positions available within the organization. A brief assessment of an applicant's interests and abilities is made before assigning the person to an interviewer. The initial screening is a sensitive personnel issue. The decision not to refer an applicant must be nondiscriminatory. As a result of the establishment of the Federal Fair Employment Practice Committee, organizations have adjusted their hiring practices and the information requested on employment applications.

The application form is designed to collect the information needed by management in referring and selecting applicants. When the application form is properly designed, it serves as an instrument to compare the applicant's qualifications with the job requirements. Information requested on the application should correlate with job success, since the application is a major resource for predicting success on the job. The designer of the application form should also realize that because applicants' backgrounds vary greatly, the level of language used should be appropriate for the vast majority. The organization must review state and federal regulations to ensure that all questions on the application are legal.

Even the most well-designed application may present information that is slightly misleading. For this reason, the most important step in the employment process is the interview. Evaluating applicants through personal interviews is a difficult task—one that is accomplished by sound interviewing methods. The personal interview (selection interview) accomplishes three major objectives:

1. It matches people and their skills to the available job.
2. It provides the applicant with information about the position and the organization.
3. It allows the interviewer to collect additional information about the applicant.

Steps in the Interview Process

Because organizations and their social environments are different, there is no foolproof method of interviewing. Generally, interviewing falls into a number of phases that may occur formally or informally, depending on the situation and the skills of the interviewer. The selection interview consists of five phases:

1. Introduction.
2. Information seeking.
3. Information giving.
4. Closure.
5. Evaluation.

Figure 1.4   What You Can and Can't Ask During an Interview

	Legal	**Not Legal**
Age	If hired, proof that at least 18 years old	Date of birth, age, proof of age
Race/Color	For ID purposes, any distinguishing physical characteristics	Race or color (hair, eyes, skin)
Name	Worked for company under different name. Previous nickname to locate records	Legally changed name Original name
Sex	None	Male/female or related questions
Religion	None (unless asking if available to work all "holidays" if applicable)	Religious affiliation, church attended, name of pastor, rabbi or priest
Residence	Present address, length of time at present address, former address and length of time there	Own or rent residence, names of people residing with you
Birthplace	If hired, provide resident alien card or birth certificate	Where applicant or parents were born
Crime Record	Convicted of a crime (job related)	Ever been arrested
Military Record	Related work experience/ training	Type of discharge
Citizenship	Citizen of USA	Citizen of what country?
National Origin	Languages applicant reads, speaks or writes fluently (job related)	Ancestry, lineage, descent, mother tongue

Gathered from the Bureau of National Affairs and other information sources of federal labor laws. Courtesy of Blaine Lester, Johnstown, PA.

During the introduction, which is the warm-up stage of the interview, the interviewer establishes rapport with the applicant. A common rapport-building tactic used by interviewers is to discuss with the applicant a topic of common interest. Small talk helps put the applicant at ease, and a friendly exchange of mutual interests leads to understanding and thus enhances the flow of information. The interviewer should ensure that interruptions are kept to a minimum so that the applicant is confident of the interviewer's complete attention.

Collecting information about the applicant is the core of the interview. Selecting the question that triggers the flow of information from the applicant is a challenge for the interviewer. This pivotal question is difficult to pose because it has to be tailored to each applicant. A common strategy used to encourage conversation is to inquire about the applicant's recent work experience.

Necessary information may be obtained by direct questioning. This approach is effective for gathering facts, but it can slow conversation if the questions are not carefully worded and clear to the applicant. Inquiries should not be put in the form of leading questions that suggest an appropriate answer, nor should they be tricky or confusing. The trust and rapport built in the interview set the tone for future employer-employee relations.

During the information-giving stage of the interview, the applicant learns about the organization, the position, the working conditions, and the employee benefits and pay. It is the responsibility of the interviewer to present important information and answer questions the applicant may have. The questions the applicant asks about the organization can reveal much about character, sense of values, and career goals.

In keeping with the objectives of the interview, the applicant's background and suitability for the position should be covered in as deliberate a fashion as is comfortable. Once the purpose of the interview has been accomplished, it should be concluded. The interview may be ended on a verbal cue; for example, the interviewer may thank the applicant for taking the time to come in and estimate when a decision will be made. Physical actions may also indicate the conclusion of an interview; the interviewer may stand and shake the applicant's hand.

Evaluation of the applicant occurs throughout the interview, and the interviewer should make mental notes of pertinent points. Immediately after the applicant has departed, a careful rating should be made. This rating may be a narrative or checklist, and it should include immediate impressions and additional information. The conclusions reached about the applicant should be documented from actual information rather than be based on conjecture.

The interviewer must determine how information about the applicant relates to interpersonal relationships on the job and suitability for the position. Most important, the information obtained should predict work performance. Comparing one applicant with others can also be helpful in reaching a decision.

Comparing the Candidates

There should be no shortage of qualified candidates for most positions, especially management positions. So, after the selection steps have been followed and two or more viable candidates remain from which to choose, consider assessing each candidate on the basis of eight criteria:

1. A strong work ethic.
2. A solid education.
3. Relationship to a mentor.
4. Experience in a quality organization.
5. Actual "hands on" experience.
6. Personal philosophy and style.
7. Results of past work experiences.
8. Initiative and opportunity seeking.*

A candidate screen or checklist will be helpful in the process of identifying the best all-around candidate. This technique is especially useful when a hiring committee is involved. With the use of a horizontal column for the names of the applicants and a series of vertical columns to list the desirable characteristics, an easy-to-read grid will allow quick reference, cross-checking, and an overall comparison of the finalists.

---

*Adapted from Heuerman, J.N. "Advice from a Head Hunter." *Healthcare Forum Journal*. July / August, 1989:37.

Reference Checks and Recommendations

Employee References

All employers have become increasingly concerned about who they hire and keep as employees due to the doctrine of negligent hiring and negligent retention. Consider the case of Donald Harvey, a hospital orderly, who in 1987 pleaded guilty to committing 24 murders in two Ohio hospitals by administering poisons to patients. The hospitals have been hit with numerous civil damage suits by relatives who contend that the employers failed to take reasonable care in assuring that Harvey was qualified to safely perform the duties of his job. Officials of the first hospital where Mr. Harvey was employed wouldn't divulge information about his job performance citing federal privacy laws and hospital personnel policies. The situation is made more chilling with the fact that courts appear to be increasingly willing to find employers liable for the malfeasance of their employees. How is an employer supposed to validly ascertain the suitability of a perspective employee? The situation is made more complicated by the Privacy Act of 1974 and the Buckley Amendment. These laws allow employees to review letters in their files. Although the law pertains to public sector employees and students, private employers reflect their concern through reference procedures that severely limit outgoing information or reference requests.

Improving Reference Validity

The standard parts of the selection process are references and recommendation letters. The purpose is to get some indication of the applicant's past behavior and job performance. For a reference check to be useful, the respondent needs to know the applicant's performance record and be competent to evaluate it. (See Figure 1.5) The respondent must also be truthful, and therein lies the major shortcoming of the reference seeking process. Because the person giving a reference fears the applicant may have access to reference information, there is a tendency to gloss over shortcomings and overemphasize good points. Removing some of the subjectivity from the reference gathering procedure will improve the validity of the reference process as a predictor of future performance. One method of job

Figure 1.5   Verifying references

What information is the most vital to verify during the reference check? These points are important:
1. Verify employment dates and positions held.
2. Check prior experience relative to the position for which the candidate applied.
3. Verify dependability, reliability, and loyalty (attendance, tardiness, task completion).
4. Ask about the candidate's ability to interact with supervisors, peers and subordinates.
5. Ask about degree of incentive or motivation.
6. Ask about daily disposition/attitude.
7. Check on communication skills.*

---

* Courtesy of Blaine Lester. Johnstown, PA.

performance verification is the job specification reference tool. In this approach, a letter of reference is constructed based on a job analysis that asks the responder to rank an applicant's performance characteristics on a weighted scale. (See Figure 1.6)

Giving References

Perspective employers should do a better job of contacting former employers when checking references. This task is made more difficult due to the current posturing of human resources managers as to reference protocols. Former employers are taking care to insulate themselves from defamation claims by former employees. In regards to reference giving:

• Put in place a written former employment reference policy; be certain that all possible contacts in the supervisory ranks understand how reference checks are to be conducted.
• Check to see that the requester of reference information has a legitimate need for the information.
• Have job applicants sign releases allowing a future employer to seek and to use reference information in order to base the employment decision.
• Get written consent from separated employees to disclose basic employment verification.
• Never blacklist a former employee for any reason.
• Take care not to offer any subjective statements that cannot be backed up in the employee's official record.
• When contacted by telephone, use a call back procedure to verify the identity of the person seeking reference information.

Figure 1.6 Sample Reference Letter for Radiographer Applicant

Dear Former Employer:
Mary Safelight has applied for a position with our hospital as a staff radiographer. She has supplied you as a reference and we need a few moments of your time to rate her effectiveness on the job. You will find below a list of statements that describe important characteristics in the job performance of a radiographer. Please rank this individual's performance by placing the appropriate number in the spaces provided.
A. Has demonstrated the ability to perform all radiographic examinations of full diagnostic quality with a minimum amount of supervision and incidence of repeat exposure.
B. Can perform most radiographic examinations in an expert manner with some supervision and guidance.
C. May be depended upon to complete assigned tasks associated with the position of radiographer.
D. Is willing to undertake difficult assignments, is anxious to learn new procedures, and is energetic in the performance of assigned duties.
E. Is always neat in appearance, is courteous, is professional in demeanor, and works well with others.
1._____ (Most describes the applicant)
2._____
3._____
4._____
5._____ (Least describes the applicant)
Comments about the applicant:

- Record who you gave any employment information to and the date it was provided.

When you're disappointed with a former employee for any reason, the temptation to share negative feelings with a perspective employer may exist. Resist that temptation to tell all. It could be a very costly slip in reference etiquette.

Employment Provisions in the ADA Protect Disabled From Discrimination

Provisions of Title I of The Americans with Disabilities Act were designed to prevent discrimination. Under the law, private employers, state and local governments, employment agencies and labor unions are prohibited from discriminating against qualified individuals with disabilities in job application procedures, hiring, firing, advancement, compensation, job training and other terms, conditions and privileges of employment.

The Act defines an individual with a disability as someone who:

- Has a physical or mental impairment that substantially limits one or more major life activities;
- Has a record of such an impairment; or
- Is regarded as having such an impairment.

A qualified employee or applicant with a disability is an individual who, with or without reasonable accommodation, can perform the essential functions of the job in question. Employers are required to make accommodations to the known disability of a qualified employee if it does not impose "undue hardship" on the operation of the business. Reasonable accommodation may include, but is not limited to the following:

- Making existing facilities used by employees readily accessible to and usable by persons with disabilities;
- Job restructuring, modifying work schedules; reassignment to a vacant position;
- Acquiring or modifying equipment or devices, adjusting or modifying examinations, training materials, or policies and providing readers or interpreters.

The ADA also prohibits employers from asking job applicants about the existence, nature or severity of a disability. During an interview, employers may only question applicants about their ability to perform the job.

Once a job offer has been made, however, the employer can require a medical exam and make the job contingent on the results. If the physician determines the disability will affect the person's ability to perform the job, the employer can rescind the offer.

Charges of employment discrimination on the basis of disability may be filed at any field office of the U.S. Equal Employment Opportunity Commission. Field officers are located in 50 cities throughout the country and are listed in most telephone directories under U.S. government.*

---

*Ellis, J. Employment Provisions in the ADA Protect Disabled from Discrimination. JMA Notes. Feb. 26, 1993, p.1.

1.5 ORIENTING THE NEW EMPLOYEE

Orientation is a process that attempts to provide a new employee with information, with skills, and with an understanding of the organization and its goals. Orientation starts the employee in the right direction towards helping that person make positive contributions in the form of good performance. Starting a new job can be a lonely and confusing event. A new job is a major change in life; the first days on the job find many people suffering from newness anxiety. A good orientation program is crucial to assisting the new employee to get started on the right course by emphasizing positive attitudes and feelings about the new job.

Purposes of Orientation

Properly done, orientation will accomplish a number of important purposes. The orientation process is a form of socialization specific to the new workplace. This socialization occurs as the new employee learns the norms, values, procedures, and performance standards that are expected in the new job. The principal purposes of new employee orientation include:

1. Reducing anxiety for the new employee.
    Fear of failure on the job is a common concern of new recruits. This is a normal fear that centers mainly on the employee's perception of his/her ability to perform new job functions. The new employee is a prime target for "hazing." A source of fun for seasoned workers is to "kid" the new employee. For instance, the old-timers will take great delight in sending a brand new student technologist to central supply for a "fallopian tube." Hazing lets the new employee know that he/she has a lot to learn; it enforces an understanding that workers are dependent upon each other for success. It is a basic lesson in working together. Hazing is a great source of anxiety to the new employee, and effective orientation alerts the new employee to this brand of workplace fun.

2. Containing the costs of start-up for the new employee.
   New employees are less efficient than an experienced worker.
   The loss of productivity can be minimized by assuring that the
   new employee is properly trained in new job duties. Give the
   new employee the tools necessary to perform the job well. Many
   technologists report examples of "being thrown to the wolves."
   The absence of written routines for various diagnostic routines
   is a common orientation blunder.
3. Minimizing employee turnover.
   Employees leave jobs when they perceive that they have become
   ineffective, unwanted, or unneeded. Turnover is high during
   this break-in period; employees say in exit interviews that they
   felt "lost in the shuffle." Not enough attention is paid to how
   new workers "feel" they are getting along. Managers react with
   shock and dismay to learn that the new employee's response to
   newness anxiety is to quit.
   The Texas Instruments Company discovered the following
   conditions during interviews with a group of new employees:
   1. Their first days on the job were anxious and disturbing.
   2. The practice of new employee initiation by peers intensified
      anxiety.
   3. The turnover of newly hired employees was caused
      primarily by anxiety.
   4. New employees were reluctant to discuss problems with
      their supervisors.
   A subsequent experiment using formal sessions of new
   employee orientation rather than the old "sink or swim" method
   improved new employee effectiveness. In general, it appeared
   that thorough and well-planned induction and orientation
   procedures were more successful.*
   Another important factor in the successful orientation process is
   preparing the organization for the new employee. Explaining the
   role to be filled by the new employee and dispelling irrational fears
   of present employees tend to make the first few weeks much easier.
4. Saving time for everyone.
   When a new employee does not receive proper orientation,
   everyone suffers. The people most likely to provide this

---

*Bittell, L. R. *What Every Supervisor Should Know*. N.Y.: McGraw Hill Book Company, 1980.

assistance are coworkers and immediate supervisors. The time spent breaking in a new employee through proper orientation saves everyone time in the end.

What the New Employee Needs to Know

During an employee's first day of work, various administrative duties associated with the induction of the new employee should be performed. Figure 1.7 describes a procedure for orienting new employees. This form should be placed in the employee's permanent personnel file after it is completed.

The first day on the job should include a discussion of the following essential facts:

1. Pay rates, pay periods, and where to pick up pay checks.
2. Hours of work, reporting and quitting time, and lunch.
3. Overtime and how it is authorized.
4. Shift differentials.
5. Time cards and location of the time clock.
6. How to report in when sick.
7. What to do when late.
8. Locations of the rest areas and washrooms.
9. Location of the employee health office.
10. Accident reporting procedures.
11. A department and hospital tour.
12. Introductions to other employees.
13. Assignment of work area.

If all of this information is explained too quickly, it can lead to confusion. Providing new employees with a copy of essential information minimizes misconceptions. Check with the new employee regularly the first few days and provide the opportunity for rediscussion of departmental rules and regulations.

What the Supervisor Needs to Know

Measures to meet the special needs of new employees are often overlooked. The supervisor should seek to make the new employee productive as soon as possible, to stimulate professional develop-

Figure 1.7 Procedure for Introducing New Employees

DEPARTMENT OF RADIOLOGY

PROCEDURE FOR INTRODUCING ALL NEW EMPLOYEES

Employee Name _____

Supervisor's Name _____

Position Title _____

1. Introduce the new employee to the individual responsible for maintaining time cards and explain the procedures for their use. _____

2. Introduce the new employee to the personnel file manager so that a permanent personnel file can be made and a name tag can be ordered. _____

3. Introduce the new employee to all department supervisors. _____

4. Inform the new employee of dress codes and personnel policies. _____

5. Introduce the new employee to the film badge coordinator and complete an application for film badge service. _____

The above named employee has completed all the processing procedures stated above.

_____
Supervisor Signature

_____
Employee Signature

ment, and to encourage constructive attitudes about work. The supervisor should set examples of constructive behavior, productive work habits, and high job satisfaction.

An effective supervisor can make the transition to a new work environment a pleasant experience by realizing that the first few days are critical for molding the motivation and the activities of a new employee. The supervisor needs to be attentive and supportive, to set clear standards of performance, and to discuss reasonable goals with the employee. Most importantly, the supervisor needs to be an acceptable role model for the employee so that appropriate behavior is reinforced daily.

Each supervisor should be encouraged to consider the answers to basic questions that new employees ask during the first days of employment. These questions usually involve specific things such as location of restrooms, dining facilities, parking areas, and transportation. Key policies and procedures also should be discussed thoroughly.

The supervisor should organize a personnel orientation plan in a notebook as an aid in structuring the new employee's first day, week, and month of employment. The notebook should contain everything the new employee needs to know in order to be effective in a position. The areas of orientation that could be outlined in the personnel orientation notebook are:

1. An overview of the orientation schedule, including check lists to ensure that the employee understands key elements of the orientation.
2. A list of personnel with similar work assignments.
3. A diagram of the physical layout of the department, with specific mention of important areas and the locations of safety materials.
4. A synopsis of pertinent policies and procedures with which a new employee should be familiar early in the orientation process.

The morale and cost-effective benefits of well-oriented employees are important concepts for supervisors to understand. An effective orientation program conveys to new employees that the organization is well managed. It also signifies that supervisors are thorough and systematic in their efforts to train employees and that they care about the special needs and interests of new employees.

Conclusion

From an administrative point of view, personnel orientation is important for three reasons. First, efficient operation of the service depends on a well-developed program of orientation. Smooth functioning depends on personnel who are familiar with the general policies of the organization, the routines of the department, and the philosophy and methods of patient care. Second, staff members must have knowledge about the department, its purposes, and organization to function smoothly within it. Third, through the orientation program the department hopes to direct the new staff member toward competent practice in a new environment.

Appendix A—New Employee Orientation

General Plant Technology and Safety*

_____ 1. Has reviewed department safety policies and procedures.
_____ 2. Has trained in the use of hazardous materials and waste management.
_____ 3. Is familiar with the Material Safety Data Sheets (MSDA) used in the work area.
_____ 4. Has trained in the proper handling of infectious waste.
_____ 5. Is familiar with the fire plan:
        _____ knows location and use of fire extinguishers.
        _____ knows evacuation routes.
        _____ is aware of hospital smoking policies.
_____ 6. Has been oriented as to proper operation of patient care equipment to be used in the job.
_____ 7. Is familiar with contingency plans in the event of utility failure.
_____ 8. Knows the location of emergency cutoffs.
_____ 9. Is familiar with the hospital disaster plan and knows his (her) role in that plan.
_____ 10. Is familiar with radiation safety procedures.

---

*JCAHO Recommended Plant/Safety Orientation

Appendix B

	MANAGEMENT
COMPANY/LOCATION	POLICY
	STANDARD

SUBJECT	DEPARTMENT	NUMBER
NEW EMPLOYEE ORIENTATION		PAGE

TITLE	DATE EFFECTIVE	DATE REVISED
NEW EMPLOYEE ORIENTATION	APPROVED BY (Signature)	APPROVED BY (Signature)

POLICY: The Radiology Department shall provide an appropriate orientation to new employees.

PURPOSE: To ensure that new personnel receive adequate training in all areas of patient care, departmental policies and physical facilities.

SPECIAL INSTRUCTIONS:

An orientation program will be used to benefit new employees entering the Radiology Department. It will consist of orienting new personnel to the physical facilities, departmental policies, and departmental procedures. This program will be used to assure that new personnel will receive adequate training in all areas of patient care provided by the hospital.

As the orientation program progresses, records will be maintained for the new employee and included in his personnel file. These records will be used to help evaluate and rate the employee's overall performance for the first three months of employment. The appropriate supervisor will be responsible for evaluating the clinical competency of the individual.

Appendix C

NEW EMPLOYEE ORIENTATION
EQUIPMENT USER TRAINING DOCUMENTATION

Name of Equipment_____

Purpose and Use of Equipment_____

Section_____

The following employee(s) have been oriented as to the safe and proper utilization of equipment used for patient care in the Department of Radiology.

_____

_____

_____

_____

The above named employee(s) perform(s) diagnostic testing and display(s) competencies necessary to produce studies such that confident professional interpretations of test results can be made.

_____
Medical Director

_____
Director

Appendix D

New Employee Check-in

Employee's Name _____ Hire Date _____

Supervisor _____ Department _____

_____ 1. Ask the employee his/her full name and the name he/she prefers to be called. Introduce him/her to the supervisor and fellow employees.

_____ 2. Discuss Mission, Vision, and Values from perspective of the department and provide examples of each.

_____ 3. Discuss the Culture necessary to support Total Quality Management.

_____ 4. Explain the shared vision of the department.

_____ 5. Discuss the work teams in the department and invite the new employee to get involved.

_____ 6. Explain the departmental organization and chain of command.

_____ 7. Provide a job description for the employee, explain the nature of the job, importance of the job, and the employee's responsibilities and duties.

_____ 8. Read dress code policy. Explain proper clothing to the employee, emphasizing departmental dress code and have the employee sign that he/she has read and understands the dress code policy.

_____ 9. Inform employee of starting and quitting time, lunch period, breaks, personal relief, and other details that apply specifically to his/her job.

_____ 10. Explain how the employee will be paid, when, where, rate of pay and method of increases.

_____ 11. Describe departmental method for handling tardiness and absenteeism.

_____ 12. Inform employee of method of drawing supplies, location of procedure and policy manuals, and other sources of information.

_____ 13. Read MSDS policies. Point out any safety hazards or hazardous material utilized within department. Read system and departmental safety policy and explain departmental safety rules.

_____ 14. Inform employee what to do in case of an accident or emergency.

_____ 15. Read system Disaster and Fire Plans. Inform employee of his/her responsibilities in carrying out the Disaster and Fire Plans.

_____ 16. Inform employee of location of locker room, lounge, restrooms, hospital entrance, exits, parking lots, and bulletin boards.

_____ 17. Show timeclock to employee and explain procedure for clocking in and out.

_____ 18. Familiarize employee with work area and any other department with which he/she will have contact.

_____ 19. Read Infection Control Policy (if applicable), and explain departmental rules to employees.

_____ 20. Indicate your willingness to help the employee, also invite questions and free communication in the future.

This orientation checklist must be completed before employee begins work.

Trainer's Name _____ Trainer's Extension _____

Signature—Employee _____ Date _____

Signature—Department Director/Manager _____ Date _____

NOTE: Items 1–7 to be completed by Department Director, manager, or immediate supervisor.

1.6 MEASURING PERFORMANCE

Why Evaluate?

Motivating employees is a difficult and complex endeavor; many behavioral scientists have written about motivation to provide a greater understanding of its dynamics. A number of popular theories of behavioral management are frequently used by health care managers. Some of these theories are briefly mentioned here. Further study in the subject of motivation may yield additional applications for radiologic employees.

The premise of most motivational theory is that human needs give rise to behavior. Therefore, the performance of employees and their relationships with others depend on their motivation. It is important to keep in mind that motives are highly individualized; that is, quite different in type, number, and intensity—depending on the individual.

There are hundreds of identifiable human needs. Attempting to know and understand all these needs would create a difficulty in applying this knowledge to the study of human behavior. Two important frameworks of needs have been developed and have become the mainstay of modern motivational theory. The first is A. H. Maslow's hierarchy of needs. Maslow's framework groups all needs into five basic categories: (1) physiological, (2) safety, (3) social, (4) esteem, and (5) self-actualization. These categories are related to each other in the form of a hierarchy that progresses in an orderly fashion. (See Figure 1.8) One category of needs is activated only after the level immediately preceding it has been satisfied. Physiological needs are regarded as primary in motivational theory because they are the most immediate of all needs. When physiological needs are satisfied, a higher level of needs emerges. These, in turn, are satisfied, and the system progresses up the hierarchy. It is essential for the manager to know that higher order needs—those of esteem and self-actualization—are most closely linked to motivation and achievement on the job.

A second major theory of motivation was developed by Frederick Herzberg. In the 1950s, Herzberg conducted a study of motivation among 200 professional and technical employees in the Pittsburgh area. The motivation of these workers was selected for study because of the continual importance these workers play in today's highly technological work environment. An analysis of survey responses

Figure 1.8   Abraham Maslow's Hierarchy of Needs

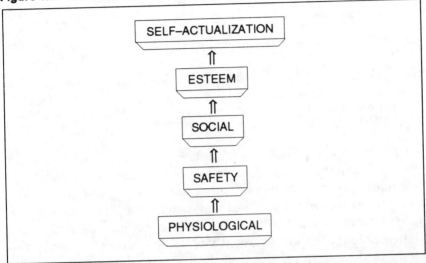

concluded that the elements of job content that gave workers the most satisfaction were motivators. Job content was defined as experiences and tasks associated with successful job performance. Maintenance factors were defined as influences related to job context, including salary, supervision and working conditions. Motivators cannot operate in the absence of maintenance factors; both must exist to maintain productivity and assure that work is a source of satisfaction. Because Herzberg's theory separates two kinds of behaviors, (i.e., satisfiers and dissatisfiers), it is called the "two factor theory."

Herzberg's theory may be compared to Maslow's hierarchy. Maslow's lower-order needs are similar to maintenance factors, and higher-order needs correspond to motivators. Figure 1.9 identifies examples of the factors that compose the motivation-maintenance model.

The motive for achievement is suggested by Maslow to be a higher-order need and by Herzberg to be a motivator that must be realized if management desires high performance from employees. Management must embrace two tasks that will help ensure personal and institutional achievement. The first is to establish an environment that provides workers with performance feedback. The second task is to formulate clear and achievable work objectives that are acceptable to both management and labor.

Figure 1.9 Herzberg's Factors That Comprise the Motivation Maintenance Model

Motivators The Job Itself	Maintenance Factors Environment
Achievement Recognition for accomplishment Challenging work Increased responsibility Growth and development	Policies and administration Supervision Working conditions Interpersonal relations Money, status, security

Performance appraisal is a method of evaluating an employee's work performance. Assessing employee performance is an important management tool in evaluating employees for staff development, training, promotion, and wage increases. The primary purpose of performance appraisal is to help the employee achieve the highest potential for achievement at work. Evaluations are an opportunity to develop a relationship with the employee that provides guidelines and support for improved performance.

Performance appraisal represents an overall view of the employee. The criteria for evaluation begin with the basic data of the job description, the degree of responsibility the job affords the individual and standards of performance. The most difficult task in establishing job performance standards is evaluating the degree to which the employee has met the standards. Therefore, written standards should determine how a job is to be done and what results are desired.

Performance appraisal may be completed by several methods. All employee assessment programs should have a standard rating system. Standards of judgment must be applied uniformly by all reviewers so that one employee's performance can be weighed equally against another.

Purposes of Performance Appraisal

The arguments, pro and con, for a formal employee performance appraisal system are heavily weighted in favor of a systematic approach, which should be in place in any organization. For hospitals, a periodic performance evaluation for each employee based on a job description is a key factor in the accreditation decision process by the Joint Commission on Accreditation of Healthcare Organizations. A formal employee performance appraisal system serves several other purposes:

- Development—It will identify which employees need more training.
- Reward—It reinforces the employee's motivation to perform more effectively via pay raises.
- Motivation—The presence of an evaluation program encourages initiative and stimulates performance.
- Legal compliance—It defends the employer for employment decisions.
- Compensation—It helps develop equity among jobs.
- Communication—It serves as the basis for ongoing discussion about job-related issues.

The Appraisal Process

An employee's personal growth, optimum performance, and professional development is strengthened by an accurate performance appraisal. In order to achieve this, performance appraisals must:

1. Be based on observable, specific, measurable, objective, job-related performance standards.
2. Be based on fair and consistent performance judgements by all managers.
3. Encourage open communication between manager and employee, to allow them to plan, evaluate, and improve performance together.
4. Tie the individual's performance, goals, and objectives to those of the department and hospital.

To provide information that can serve the organization's goals and that can comply with the law, a performance evaluation system must provide accurate and reliable information. The factors upon which an employee is evaluated are called the "criteria of evaluation." The criteria used are critical in effective performance evaluation systems and should be based on four major characteristics of effectiveness:

1. **Relevant**—valid measures closely related to job duties.
2. **Unbiased**—based on the work performed, not the person performing the work.

3. **Significant**—directly related to department goals.
4. **Practical**—measurable and efficient.

Figure 1.10 is a sample worksheet used to collect supporting information for the performance appraisal.

There are several ways that one can go about collecting the data for measuring an individual's performance:

1. Observation of work behaviors: This would be firsthand observations by the appraiser of the things that the employee does or does not do relevant to what should be done. This could be in the form of Direct Observations (quantified) or Supervisory Observations (discretionary judgment of overall work behavior).
2. Observation of the products of behavior: This refers to the outcomes of an employee's actions, the additions or deletions in the work because of the behavior. The outcome would be a

Figure 1.10

EVALUATION WORKSHEET		
MAJOR DUTIES	PERFORMANCE STANDARD	RATING* 4 3 2 1
1)_____		
2)_____		
3)_____		
4)_____		
5)_____		
6)_____		

*4 = Less than 50% of time meets standard
3 = 50–75% of time meets standard
2 = 76–89% of time meets standard
1 = 90% or more of time meets standard

completed task or service that could be examined for quality or appropriate quantity produced over time.

3. Observation of extended consequences of behavior: This refers to consequences of the actions of the individual that are removed from the immediate result and that *may be reported by a third party*, such as complaints by someone about the way this individual performs, added costs of operations, equipment downtime, and so forth.

4. Observation of goal achievement: This refers to the approximation of performance outcomes as related to previously identified and specified goals. These are usually quantifiable as specific measurable changes in the work within a time framework and related to observations in 1, 2, and 3. What is measured under this differs from observations 1, 2, and 3 only in the way it is targeted in advance.

The Appraisal Interview

A successful appraisal interview should be well planned in advance. The following suggestions are designed to reduce arbitrariness and to improve the clarity of the interaction between supervisor and the employee.

It is the supervisor's responsibility to speak clearly, to listen carefully, and to set a respectful tone.

1. Prepare for the session in advance and be ready to discuss the employee's performance against the job criteria.

2. Put the employee at ease and make it clear that performance appraisal is not a disciplinary action.

3. Share the time for the session equally so that the employee has an opportunity to discuss the evaluation.

4. Use facts; evidence must be available to document any claims.

5. Begin and conclude with positive remarks; sandwich performance shortcomings between other positive points.

6. Balance the amount of information given to the employee; guard against overwhelming the employee with too much information.

7. Focus on future objectives and how the employee can accomplish these objectives.

1.7 COUNSELING THE INEFFECTIVE EMPLOYEE

Managers will inevitably be faced with the necessity of telling an employee in clear terms that his or her behavior or job performance needs improvement. The way you conduct the interview will determine whether your advice can help the employee make the transition to improved performance. During this disciplinary interview, there are several elements that will influence the success of the exercise. They are appropriate scheduling, the right setting, careful preparation, and a plan of action.

Scheduling the Session

The best time of day for counseling is early in the morning. Conducting the counseling the first thing in the morning will allow plenty of time to complete your discussions; a disciplinary action should never be hurried. It also gives you the remainder of the day to work with the employee and to let him know that you accept him as a person, even though you object to his behavior. This also removes some of the punitive aspects of the counseling, and the employee will feel less chastened. Should the employee wish to have further discussion about the counseling, the remainder of the day is available for that purpose. If you schedule the interview close to lunch time, the employee will probably unload anger on the sympathetic ears of coworkers. There is a significant risk that your disgruntled employee will then infect your other subordinates with feelings of tension and anger. At least with a counseling session scheduled early in the day, the rest of the morning may serve to reduce your employee's defensiveness.

Choosing the Right Setting

Conduct your counseling session in a private place where you will not be interrupted. Your employee will be very anxious and the slightest distractions will increase his tension. Remember that this attempt to take corrective action for poor performance is a very private affair between you and the employee. Public chastisement humiliates the employee and disturbs coworkers.

The counseling interview is not a social occasion and should not be attempted over lunch or a rest break. No one likes to be called to the boss's office; there is a negative connotation to such a summons. Usually, the manager's office is the only available place to conduct the interview, although to use the subordinate's private office is also appropriate. In fact, the manager enjoys a greater flexibility as to how to end the interview if it occurs in an office other than his own; he can simply leave when he is finished. This option helps short circuit a subordinate's attempt to be resistant to the counseling process with a standoff.

Preparing for the Counseling Interview

Sitting down with an employee to discuss a performance problem is never an impromptu activity. In fact, by the time it is necessary to take such a disciplinary action, the employee has already received a warning that his performance or behavior is not meeting standards. You will need objective evidence of the problem. Careful documentation of your case is essential considering today's antidiscrimination laws.

During your discussion of the employee's performance, concentrate on the one critical issue to resolve and avoid preparing a "laundry list" of problems and complaints. Counseling an employee in more than one major deficiency is usually not productive. The attention needs to be focused in order to change the problem behavior. Some managers make the mistake of overwhelming the employee with a long list of errors and mistakes. To the employee, this appears to be a grudge session, and the result is a resentful employee whose performance probably won't improve. There are several guidelines that can help the manager have a constructive session with an ineffective performer.

1. Consider the causes. Determine if personal problems are playing a role in the poor performance. Listen to the employee, talk to co-workers, and observe the employee at work.
2. Investigate other reasons for poor performance. If personal problems are not the cause of the performance deficiencies,

examine other factors such as lack of skill or training, poor effort, or situational circumstances out of the employee's control.

3. Conduct a professional interview. The counseling interview needs to be private; public criticism is always negative. Emphasize job-related performance concerns in a constructive manner. Let the employee give his side of the story and be a good listener. Concentrate on the problem and avoid personal criticism that will leave the other person feeling defeated and unworthy.

4. Make the discipline clear. Describe the disciplinary steps to be taken in specific terms and state the timetable in which you expect performance to improve. Be certain that the employee understands the discipline and what the expected improvement must be.

Design a Plan of Action

The disciplinary interview is a serious part of the management job; however, it is difficult for many managers to conduct such interviews and equally difficult for them to plan. A constructive disciplinary interview will play an important role in converting an ineffective performer into a productive member of the organization. A way to reduce your stress at having to counsel a subordinate is to develop a plan of action for the counseling session. A plan of operation for the interview is found in figure 1.11.

In summary, discipline is one of the most challenging aspects of a manager's job. Ineffective performance may be the result of skill, job, or motivational climate factors. All of these factors must be weighed

Figure 1.11 Ten Steps in the Counseling Sequence

1. Problem statement.
2. Agreement on the deficiency.
3. Listening.
4. Extenuating circumstances.
5. Referral (if necessary).
6. Finding a desirable alternative behavior.
7. Agreement on that alternative behavior.
8. Designing a corrective action plan.
9. Gaining the employee's complete understanding and cooperation.
10. Further action.

in a systematic approach of investigating and addressing performance problems.

Appendix A

Employee Performance Deterioration

Visible Signs

- [ ] Often Tardy (Especially After Lunch)
- [ ] Leaves Job Early
- [ ] Absent (Plausible Reasons)
- [ ] Frequent Days Off for Vague Ailments
- [ ] Implausible Excuses
- [ ] Unpredictable, Prolonged Absences
- [ ] Complains of Not Feeling Well
- [ ] Lies—When Truth Would Serve
- [ ] Fellow Workers Complain
- [ ] Behavior Becomes Inconsistent
- [ ] Statements Become Unreliable
- [ ] Begins To Avoid Former Associates
- [ ] Borrows Money From Coworkers
- [ ] Hospitalized More Than Average
- [ ] Frequent Minor Injuries—On/Off Job
- [ ] Unreasonable Resentments
- [ ] Grandiose, Aggressive Behavior
- [ ] Domestic Problems Interfere with Job
- [ ] Loss of Values
- [ ] Financial Problems, Garnishment
- [ ] Refuses to Discuss Problems
- [ ] Spasmodic Work Pace—Mistakes
- [ ] Low Concentration Ability—Wanders
- [ ] Job Performance Below Expectation Level
- [ ] Drinking/Drug Using On the Job
- [ ] Frequently Undependable
- [ ] Visible Physical Deterioration
- [ ] Serious Family Problems/Divorce
- [ ] Repeatedly Inconsistent
- [ ] Incompetent

Appendix B

*Changing the Distrust Cycle**

Could you have a productive marriage if each party constantly suspected the other's motives?

It's the same in business. Most problems between managers and employees stem from *mistrust*. Each party assumes the others operate from self-interest, achieving their goals at its expense.

For instance, a front-line employee said, "They put out rumors there will be layoffs just to get people to work harder."

The firm's owner said, "I gave up on trying to treat people equally. Some are what I call 'workers'—they only want to put in their time and no more. Why should I treat them special?"

These individuals distrust each other, and each believes the other will subvert fair treatment of customers or themselves for self-interest.

So their relationship gradually deteriorates. Each new policy or organizational change causes a fresh outbreak of tension.

Here is how a distrust cycle works:

1. **Negative assumptions.** A manager believes employees will "test" his policies to "see how far they can go." A worker is a few minutes late to work twice that week.
2. **Self-protective behavior.** The manager suspects the employee is testing the attendance policy. At a staff meeting, he say he will not tolerate tardiness.
3. **Observed aggressive behavior.** The manager's comments take the employee by surprise. Feeling humiliated before her peers, she becomes angry.
4. **Reinforced negative assumptions.** The employee decides her boss is insecure and is "power-tripping," that he is insensitive ("He didn't even ask me why I was late") and unfair to her. She fears he will put her tardiness in an upcoming performance appraisal to make her toe the mark.
5. **Self-protective behavior.** The employee nervously confronts the manager, demanding to know how many minutes constitute lateness.
6. **Observed defensive behavior.** The manager feels put on the spot with a nit-picking, defensive question.

7. **Reinforced negative assumptions.** The manager feels vindicated in his initial belief: that employees will test decisions and policies and must be monitored for compliance.

This cycle, which recurs at all levels of organizations and on many different issues, stems from *negative assumptions.*

But an alternate cycle can emerge from *positive* beliefs. If people presume they can *trust* one another, strong bonds develop. Suppose managers assume *employees:*

- Want to take responsibility;
- Care about their work;
- Take the larger view of things;
- Own up to their mistakes;
- Can understand budgetary and political realities;
- Don't focus only on their rights;
- Are intrinsically honest.

Suppose workers think *managers:*

- Care about personal issues;
- Prefer solving problems with them;
- Will use their power for organization, not private, ends;
- Want to keep the workload fair;
- Take pride in operating squarely;
- Don't think they are better than their employees;
- Consider retaliation a weakness.

These assumptions are truer than many managers and employees believe. Often people make *positive* assumptions about *themselves* but *negative* ones about the *other* side. Each group believes the other wants different things in situations where both value the same things.

Distrust breeds regulations; trust breeds relationships.

Human connections matter more than organizational ones. Things get done more because of relationships, not clear job descriptions. Organizational structures are no substitute for trust and opportunity.

---

*Kathleen Ryan and Daniel Oestreich, *Driving Fear Out of the Workplace*, Jossey-Bass, 350 Sansome St., San Francisco, CA 94104. As adapted by the Pryor Report Vol 19(1):8, 1993

1.8 CLINICAL LADDERS

The retention of skilled healthcare workers concerns every clinical provider in the nation. Not only is there a shortage of qualified personnel in most healthcare disciplines, but also the competition for tenured practitioners among hospitals and clinics in the same service area intensifies the seriousness of retention strategies. The seasoned employee is a valuable resource. In order to retain that employee, an attractive package of benefits and opportunities for job enrichment needs to be put into place. Not all employees seek promotion through the traditional routes of supervision; many choose to remain clinicians and want to be rewarded for continued increasing clinical competence. A reward system for those who remain in full-time patient care is the clinical ladder concept.

Clinical Ladder Defined

A clinical ladder program is a system that uses voluntary promotions as a means to recognize increased skills and responsibility of those employees who choose to remain in direct clinical practice. The goal of management in endorsing the clinical ladder concept is to provide a work environment that challenges professional growth and recognizes excellence in clinical practice. For employees it is a way to advance in salary and in prestige without taking the traditional routes of advancement through educational or supervisory positions. A narrow managerial hierarchy in most radiology departments, combined with supervisory positions held by long-time personnel with no reason to move, leave the advancement-minded employee with only one option, moving to another institution. With a goal of retaining personnel with greater clinical skills, the clinical ladder offers an ideal avenue for employees to be rewarded for job knowledge and additional responsibilities without placing the employee in a supervisory role. See figure 1.12 for questions and answers about clinical ladders.

Figure 1.12 Clinical Ladders—Question and Answers

1. What is the clinical ladder?

The clinical ladder is a system that rewards and recognizes clinical skills and expertise demonstrated by an employee. The goal is to encourage and motivate employees by measuring job satisfaction, responsibility, and confidence during advancement through the various levels of the clinical ladder.

2. What is the difference between a clinical ladder and a career ladder?

Clinical ladder is a term used to describe a system that recognizes and rewards employees who continue to practice clinical skills. A clinical ladder is a hierarchy of criteria intended to provide a means of evaluation and/or development of employees providing direct patient care. In contrast, a *career ladder* is intended to facilitate advancement to different job categories.

3. Why establish a clinical ladder system?

A clinical ladder challenges employees to demonstrate a high level of standards and excel in their clinical area. It will recognize their efforts and expertise and provide them with an avenue of promotion within the system.

4. How many levels will there be?

There are a number of attainable levels. For example, level I is the beginning or entry level. The number of levels available in a clinical ladder system is dictated by the design of that system. Most clinical ladder systems operate with four levels.

5. What is the difference between levels?

With each level achieved, the employee is expected to have obtained and be able to demonstrate increasing levels of responsibility, clinical/technical knowledge and expertise.

6. How will educational background affect advancement?

Continuing education credits are required for all levels of advancement. Advanced educational degrees, however, are not required but can be used to advance in the clinical ladder. If an employee has obtained a degree prior to entering the clinical ladder, it can be used for the purpose of qualifying that employee for advancement or advanced standing.

7. What happens if the employee has twenty years of experience?

The clinical ladder system recognizes longevity and dedication as qualities in an employee that can be used for purposes of advancement in the clinical ladder.

8. What if an employee believes he is ready for a higher level on the clinical ladder but lacks the years of clinical experience necessary for advancement to that level?

Application criteria must be met prior to applying for advancement. Years of experience are necessary and important in developing the skills and knowledge necessary to achieve higher levels.

9. Does previous experience with other employers count towards advancement in the clinical ladder?

Yes, initial placement occurs at hire and the appropriate level is awarded at that time.

Figure 1.12 (Continued)   Clinical Ladders—Question and Answers

---

10. Must all employees participate in the clinical ladder?
   No one is obligated or penalized for not participating in the clinical ladder system. It is designed for those employees who demonstrate and want to be recognized for their exceptional clinical/technical skills.

11. Will part-time status affect an application for clinical advancement?
   Part-time employees can advance through the clinical ladder the same as full-time workers.

12. Is education mandatory?
   Educational degrees are not required for advancement in the clinical ladder system. However, every employee in a clinical advancement track must have the required CEUs to progress in levels.

How It Works

At Pitt County Memorial Hospital (PCMH), Greenville, North Carolina, Sandra Harrison, Administrator of Radiology Services, uses a clinical ladder process introduced in 1972. It has been constantly refined up to the point in 1991 where it is described in some detail in the literature.*

At PCMH, a voluntary promotion system recognizes professionals with advanced clinical knowledge and skills and allows these clinicians to assume enhanced professional roles with increased authority and responsibility. The PCMH program has established four levels of professional practice. Responsibility increases and corresponds to the scope of professional functioning needed at the prescribed level. There are specific behaviors expected at each level; they are based on criteria found in five broad areas of professional activity:

1. Education.
2. Leadership.
3. Professional practice.
4. Quality assurance.
5. Special projects/research.

---

*Davis, D., et al. "Meeting the Challenge—A Multidisciplinary Clinical Ladder Program." *Administrative Radiology*.10:1 (16-20)91.

Eligibility for Advancement

There are specific eligibility requirements for promotion in a clinical ladder. See figure 1.13 for an example of a techinical clinical ladder outline. Those requirements could involve a specific length of service at a current level, clinical competence as evidenced by performance reviews and continuing education activities. Eligibility requirements established at PCMH are as follows:

A. Requirements for a Level I professional to advance to a Level II professional:
   1. Must be a regular full-time or part-time Clinical Services professional.
   2. Must be a Level I professional at PCMH for six months or more and have at least one year of experience in area of concentration.
   3. Three evaluations that indicate that the applicant performs Level II behavior at a satisfactory level or above:
      a. Self-evaluation.
      b. Peer evaluation by Level II professional, if available.
      c. Supervisor/Manager evaluation.
   4. Must have completed yearly evaluation with department manager's review and be evaluated as being meritorious in all five categories.
   5. Evidence of required special project(s) being planned and implemented successfully.
B. Requirements for promotion from Level II to Level III:
   1. Must be a regular full-time or part-time Clinical Services professional.
   2. Must have at least one year experience at PCMH in Level II.
   3. Three evaluations that indicate the applicant performs Level III behaviors at a satisfactory level or above:
      a. Self-evaluation.
      b. Peer evaluation by a Level III, if available.
      c. Supervisor/Manager evaluation.
   4. Must have completed yearly evaluation with department manager's review and be evaluated as being meritorious.

Figure 1.13   Technical Clinical Ladder

Basic Requirements

Level I: RT I

- Current state licensure
- 1-2 years current clinical experience
- Completion of an appropriate specific orientation program
- Must be a registered technologist (ARRT) with a minimum of a diploma or ASD
- Must meet all performance standards and adhere to the policies and procedures specific to the section assigned
- Will have had no disciplinary actions within the previous twelve month period

Level II: RT II

- Meets, maintains and exceeds all requirements for Level I
- Must have 3-5 years of current clinical experience
- Meets and maintains all the standard requirements necessary to qualify for a level II employee
- Must have earned 20 contact hours of CEU in the past year
- Will have had no disciplinary actions within the previous twelve month period

Level III: RT III

- Meets, maintains and exceeds all requirements for Level II
- Must have 6-8 years of current clinical experience
- Meets and maintains all the standard requirements necessary to qualify for a level III employee
- Must have earned 20 contact hours of CEU in the past year
- Will have had no disciplinary actions within the previous twelve month period

Level IV: RT IV

- Meets, maintains and exceeds all requirements for Level III
- Must have 9 or more years of current clinical experience
- Must have earned 30 contact hours of CEU in the past year
- Will have had no disciplinary actions within the previous twelve month period

5. Evidence of required special project(s) being planned and implemented successfully.

C. Requirements for promotion from Level III to Level IV:

1. Must be a regular full-time or part-time Clinical Services professional.

2. Must have at least one year experience at PCMH in Level III.

3. Three evaluations that indicate the applicant performs Level IV behaviors at a satisfactory level or above:

a. Self-evaluation.

b. Peer evaluation by a Level IV, if available.

c. Supervisor/Leadership evaluation.

4. Must have completed yearly evaluation as being meritorious.
5. Evidence of required special project(s) being planned and implemented successfully.

Professional Practice Standards

Gail Nielsen et al. in their career strategies task force report* stated that professional practice standards include most of the technical and professional aspects of the work performance of technologists and sonographers. Criteria-based personnel evaluations of today spell out the requirements of measurable performance and expectations. When technical skills are delineated into advancement programs, each progressive step or level requires either additional criteria be incorporated into work responsibilities, or a greater degree of skill, intensity, or independence be required in the performance of the tasks.

An example of increased responsibility or independence is the performance of routine diagnostic procedures by a level I radiologic technologist compared with the performance for special procedures or surgical procedures by a level II or III technologist.

Professional practice standards, as differentiated from educational or scholarly standards, are the standards of performance for the duties of applying specific techniques, protocols and patient care functions. These standards are those functions that are required of credentialed technologists and sonographers to perform imaging and therapy procedures. Following are some of the standards identified through review of available advancement programs.

- Demonstrates thorough familiarity with all aspects of each procedure.
- Performs routine imaging exams.
- Performs minor special procedures.
- Performs special diagnostic procedures.
- Performs invasive therapeutic procedures.
- Applies appropriate radiation safety measures.
- Applies working knowledge of clerical systems.

---

*"Advancement Programs in the Workplace." Summit on Manpower. Sudbury, MA. May, 1992, p. 6.

- Performs maximum procedures per day.
- Performs unsupervised procedures independently.
- Takes call.
- Maximizes efficient materials utilization.
- Maintains sterile technique.
- Adheres to established policies, procedures, and guidelines.
- Completes certification for venipuncture.
- Completes mandatory education programs.
- Attends minimum number of department meetings,
- Attends minimum number of inservices annually.
- Attends minimum number of local professional society meetings.
- Attends periodic training to update special skills.
- Applies emergency and resuscitative procedures effectively.
- Maintains license or permit to practice as required.
- Maintains minimum education hours annually in specialty areas.
- Keeps supervisors informed of problems and issues.

Benefits

Improved recruitment and retention is the chief benefit of a clinical ladder program. Morale among current employees rises as it becomes evident that a chance for advancement exists for all employees. Obviously, more satisfied employees remain on the job and contribute to a work force which is richer in job knowledge and clinical experience. In the final analysis, clinical ladders afford employees the opportunity to advance as clinicians only, giving the much relied upon clinical practitioner a new pride and some individual control over personal advancement in a profession.

Appendix A

*GLOSSARY**

Advancement The forward or upward progress of an individual through a promotion to greater responsibility, authority or pay.

---

* From: "Advancement Programs in the Workplace." Summit on Manpower. Sudbury, MA. May, 1992, p. 23.

Advancement Program A formal, written guideline defining how workers can advance to positions of higher rank, importance, or pay (e.g., career ladders).

FTEs (Full-time equivalent) The number of full-time equivalents is determined by dividing the total hours worked annually by the total possible hours of one employee (e.g., 2080 hours).

Pay grades Levels of pay defined in the workplace for specific job functions or job descriptions.

Peer Review Process of employees commenting on or rating the performance of coworkers.

Quality Improvement The ongoing process of improving the ways an institution meets and exceeds its customers' expectations.

Quality Assurance Activities of the hospital designed to access and improve the quality of patient care. Reference: *Accreditation Manual for Hospital.* Joint Commission on the Accreditation of Healthcare Organizations, 1992 edition.

Quality Control In radiology, generally refers to monitoring operations against standards for technical specifications for equipment operations and image production.

Registry National credentialing of health professionals.

Multicredentialed Individuals who are certified or licenced in two or more disciplines and may have completed two or more accredited educational programs.

Multicompetent Individuals who hold credentials or licensure in one discipline and have skills in areas outside of that discipline. The term is often incorrectly used to define multicredentialed individuals.

Specialties Specialized areas of imaging in or related to radiology such as ultrasound, nuclear medicine, computed tomography, magnetic resonance, mammography.

Team Process The working together of a group of people to review and improve the processes of producing a product or service.

Turnover Rate at which new workers are hired to replace those who leave or are dismissed from a workplace.

Appendix B

Levels of Responsibility for a Technical Position

Level 1	Level II	Level III
Professional Practice Standards		
1. Observes policies and procedures	Contributes to development of policies and procedures	Writes policies and procedures
2. Attends inservices as directed	Assists in presenting inservices, makes report annually	Develops and presents classes for new concepts or techniques
3. Performs routine procedures	Performs specialized procedures 50% of work time	Performs specialized procedures 80% of work time
4. Effectively applies emergency and resuscitative procedures	Maintains supplies and equipment for emergency care	Instructs new hires in use and maintenance of emergency supplies and equipment
Education		
1. Holds a certificate from an AMA accredited program	Holds an associate degree in a related field	Holds a baccalaureate degree in a related field
Leadership		
1. Mentors students	Supervises students	Teaches students
2. Collects statistical data as required	Reports statistics monthly	Analyzes statistics and recommends action
3. Participates in team projects	Leads team projects	Designs and initiates team projects
4. Uses supplies effectively without waste	Maintains supply inventories	Orders supplies for a given section or department
5. Serves as a marketing agent through superior patient interaction	Recommends marketing opportunities	Writes or directs marketing proposals
Quality Improvement		
1. Collects quality improvement data as required	Tabulates and reports monthly/quarterly quality improvement data	Analyzes monthly/quarterly quality improvement reports and recommends action

From: "Advancement Programs in the Workplace." Summit on Manpower. Sudbury, MA. May, 1992, p. 9.

2. Performs quality control procedures as prescribed	Reviews quality control standards	Supervises quality control protocols
3. Reports equipment failures and abnormalities promptly	Trouble shoots equipment failures; notifies supervisor	Trouble shoots equipment failures, documents and calls for service
4. Follows guidelines for reducing costs and improving quality	Suggests potential costs savings or improvements in quality	Identifies cost saving procedures and reviews potential process improvements

Scholarly Activities

1. Holds membership in professional society	Attends professional society meetings	Contributes to professional society activities (e.g., holds office or chairs committee)
2. Keeps abreast of professional publications; demonstrates familiarity with new concepts and techniques	Presents reports or published articles to department meetings twice annually	Publishes professional articles annually
3. Keeps abreast of new research through professional journals	Assists in research projects	Writes grants, initiates research

1.9 MANAGING PRODUCTIVITY

Productivity measurement has rapidly gained a prominent place in the contemporary vocabulary of hospital administrators. Productivity, simply stated, is the continual monitoring, measuring, and improving of healthcare delivery. It matches available labor hours with demand for services while containing the costs of doing business. Productivity measurement determines how much and how well healthcare is provided in a given setting.

Closely associated with productivity are effectiveness and efficiency. Effectiveness describes the ability to produce desired results from an activity. Efficiency is simply a comparison of return on investment; that is, the ratio of output to input per unit. The goal of measuring productivity is to meet the current demand for cost containment while still maintaining high-quality patient care.

Productivity in radiology usually centers around the yield of examinations per technical hour; but behind the concept of productivity are people (i.e., workers, supervisors and managers) who perform the work that delivers the service. Assuming the presence of good equipment and working facilities, productivity is a function of employees' abilities and motivation to perform well. Effective communication and encouragement of employee participation in relevant management decisions aid in the success of programs designed to improve productivity. The absence of employee participation in planning and designing such measures generally has a negative effect on productivity. A lack of acceptance and unwillingness to adopt new ideas, such as revised work schedules and improved patient flow measures, can be avoided with employee input into plans for change. In fact, employees offer new insight into old problems because they are intimately acquainted with the work process and will often suggest great solutions.

Managing and controlling input and output levels for improving productivity requires a method of measuring the work load. It is necessary to establish reporting procedures to aid in work measurement. The initial measurement of output in radiology departments is relatively simple because the radiologic examination is a quantitative product. In fact, for years radiology supervisors have been counting the procedures that have formed the criteria for estimations about personnel needs, equipment acquisitions, and department size. However, a productivity management program entails more than a simple count of the procedures performed in the department. The organization of reporting systems to monitor procedures and productivity levels yields utilization data and provides a statistical base for planning.

Standardizing Work Load

The procedure count, although a useful number, is not a very accurate indicator of radiologic activity. It does not consider the diversity of procedures, the complexity of the studies, and the variances in the time required to perform different procedures.

Measuring productivity with the use of work units, rather than with the procedure count, is a more accurate method of monitoring activity. The work unit is a more usable indicator because it includes adjustments for the degree of difficulty of various radiographic examinations. The California Medical Association developed relative value studies in the 1960s to assist physicians in structuring their professional charges. A method to record work load in clinical laboratories was developed by the College of American Pathologists in 1970. Other time measurement tools for radiologic procedures are currently available, such as the Canadian Workload Measurement System, the Harvard RVS System, and RADWORKS marketed by the American Healthcare Radiology managers.

The Relative Value

The relative value unit method of measuring productivity relates output to the amount of time required to perform an examination. Output, then, can be assigned a relative value after required technical staff time is accurately computed. The basic system correlates each individual radiographic examination to a base unit of time. The chest radiographic examination, for example, is a typical base unit for computations in relative value scales. A chest radiograph takes the least time to perform—three to five minutes. An examination that requires five minutes to perform would therefore have a relative value of one. A chest examination would be assigned a relative value unit of one, where one RVU equals five minutes. Examinations are rated in multiples of five minutes. For example, examinations that require 20 minutes of technical employee time are assigned a relative value of four.

During a 24-hour period, a piece of radiographic equipment is considered available for a maximum of 288 RVUs (24 hours x 12 RVUs/hr). Administrators usually want to measure the productivity of the radiology department during peak operating times. During an eight-hour shift, a radiographic room is available for 96 RVUs (12 RVUs x 8 hrs). The percentage of personnel utilization is calculated by dividing the actual RVUs expended by the potential RVUs. For example:

Room Utilization (8 Hours)

10 upper GI series	x	4 RVUs each	=	40 RVUs
11 chest examinations	x	1 RVU each	=	11 RVUs
1 lumbar spine	x	3 RVUs each	=	3 RVUs
2 IVP examinations	x	12 RVUs each	=	24 RVUs
			TOTAL	78 RVUs

78 actual RVUs
96 potential RVUs (8 hrs x 12 RVUs/hr) = 81% utilization rate.

The percentage of personnel utilization is calculated by dividing the number of work hours into the number of RVUs accomplished during a time span. For example:

Personnel Utilization (an 8 hr period involving 2 persons assigned to an examining room)

8 upper GI series	x	4 RVUs each	=	32 RVUs
13 chest examinations	x	1 RVU each	=	13 RVUs
2 cervical spines	x	3 RVUs each	=	6 RVUs
1 T-tube cholangiogram	x	8 RVUs each	=	8 RVUs
1 IVP	x	12 RVUs each	=	12 RVUs
1 air-contrast colon	x	12 RVUs each	=	12 RVUs
			TOTAL	83 RVUs

83 actual RVUs
192 potential RVUs (16 work hrs x 12 RVUs/hr) = 43% personnel utilization.

The ancillary staff in radiology also can be monitored with relative-value-based analysis of activity. The efficiency of transportation assistants is a universal challenge for the radiology manager. Escorting patients to and from the radiology department is an activity that does not differ significantly in the time required. On the average, 20 minutes is an adequate time for round-trip transportation of hospitalized patients. The relative value of one round-trip escort for the transportation assistant is assigned an RVU of four. The transportation assistant, therefore, should be able to escort three patients per hour for a total of twenty-four per day. A radiology department that requires ninety-six inpatients transported per day will utilize four full-time transportation assistants:

12 potential RVUs = 3 patient trips/hour
3 patient trips/hour x 8 hours = 24 patient trips/day
24 patient trips x 4 transportation assistants = 96 patient trips

Work Measurement Methodology

In dealing with the immediate problem of rising healthcare costs, it must be understood that effective cost containment depends on increased productivity. Wages and benefits are nearly 60 percent of typical hospital costs; therefore, more creative management of employee productivity will have a substantial impact on cost containment measures. A productivity enhancement program will result in a more efficient operation; that is, improved staffing and cost savings.

Time studies are the most popular method of measuring work, and they enable the development of valid work standards. The relative value system previously described is derived from a representative average of information collected during actual practice. Figure 1.14 is an example of relative value units assigned to typical radiologic examinations. A comprehensive list of radiologic examinations and their respective value units is essential to any radiology department that chooses to measure productivity by the relative-value unit system. Establishing relative-value units is highly individualized and depends on the characteristics of the department. The complexity of the examination, the patients, and the type of hospital are some of the deciding characteristics.

Determining the actual times for specific examinations is crucial for accurate formulation of RVUs. The RVU is a product of averaging, so a representative number of each examination type should be surveyed before assigning units.

Productivity and People

Improved productivity depends upon the highest level of utilization of each person working in the department. The full-utilization theory is a philosophy that the radiology manager must adopt to achieve goals of effectiveness, efficiency, and economy. The full-utilization philosophy is based on the marriage of two fundamental principles. First, the objectives of the organization are accomplished through the people who work there. Second, within the context of the objectives of the organization, the opportunity exists for the employee to accomplish personal goals.

Figure 1.14   Relative Value Units for Selected Radiologic Procedures

PROCEDURE	AVERAGE TIME (Min)	RVU*
Abdomen	5	1
Angiocardiography	100	20
Ankle	5	1
Breast (Bilateral)	30	6
Chest	5	1
Cholangiogram (T-Tube)	40	8
Cerebral Angiogram (Unilateral)	60	12
Facial Bones	15	3
Lumbar Spines	20	4
Mandible	15	3
Paranasal Sinuses	20	4
Skull	15	3
Sternum	15	3
Thoracic Spines	10	2

*Divide average time by 5

The success of a productivity improvement program stems from properly managing the human assets of an organization. Some key points to emphasize in employee relations that are related to productivity and job satisfaction are:

1. Employees should participate in concerns for increased productivity. Good communication and employee participation in planning and implementing productivity measures will help with acceptance of the program and minimize misconceptions.
2. Technological changes and the resultant effect on job content should be discussed. In the earlier part of this century, science and technology were synonymous with progress. But there is recent concern that the environment and quality of life are endangered by unrestricted technological development. Employees are reluctant to accept change for the sake of improved technology if their jobs may be threatened.
3. A sound performance appraisal system should be initiated, allowing management the opportunity to reinforce good performance and offer constructive discussion about improving

performance. The performance evaluation interview is a good opportunity for the employee to participate in establishing goals and determining ways to measure when those goals have been accomplished.

4. Employees who possess abilities that can be put to maximum use by the department should be selected. It is also important that these individuals be placed in situations that meet their own needs and expectations. Highly motivated radiographers, with expertise in a technical aspect of radiologic care, will quickly become disenchanted if they are not given the opportunity to exercise their talents with challenging work.

5. Working conditions should be conducive to maintaining good morale. Employees will be proud to be part of a pleasant working environment, with clean and attractive surroundings that complement professional competence.

6. The organizational structure of the department should be such that responsibility for operations is spread among a number of employees. Supervisors should take every opportunity to give subordinates a chance to exhibit initiative and ingenuity.

7. Job content needs to be reviewed continually to keep the interest and satisfaction of employees high. Techniques such as job rotation, job sharing and job enrichment are ways to prevent employees from settling into a routine rather than highly productive behavior.

8. Employee training should be designed not only to maintain continuing competence, but also to promote both lateral and upward mobility. Supervisory training should emphasize theories of motivational dynamics and interpersonal relations skills.

9. Financial incentives will help motivate employees toward better job performance. Compensation should be set at a rate that is commensurate with the level of work performed and comparable to similar compensation scales in the community.

10. Different leadership styles will be necessary for different situations and employees. Select supervisory personnel who have the required skills and knowledge to create situations in which employees can satisfy the productivity objectives of management and still feel that their personal needs are met.

1.10 RECRUITING AND RETAINING PROFESSIONAL STAFF

The recruitment, selection, and retention of personnel is a critical operational responsibility for radiology managers. Selection is the procedure that culminates with securing a successful employee from an applicant pool. Personnel decisions depend on correspondence among individuals, work personalities, and the work environment. An understanding of organizational behavior—the study and application of information about human behavior at work—is the foundation on which modern human resources administration is based.

In the 1990s, changes in human and managerial technology and philosophy are causing organizations to review their functions and to provide for "quality of work life." The need to make the most of human potential is reflected in these changes and is a challenge to managers. Changes in the workplace are attributed to: 1) understanding of people based on knowledge of human needs; 2)managing people with humanistic and democratic ideals; and 3) appreciating the mechanism of power through collaboration and reason. Quality of work life comprises two related conditions. First, the decision to work is based on how a job meets the individual's personal needs. Second, human dignity is maintained by organizing work in a fashion that is meaningful to the individual and still meets the objectives of the organization.

An organization exists when people and technology are directed toward a common end. The *people*, and the *technology* they practice, work within a *structure*, usually a well-defined hierarchy. These three elements are affected by external forces—the environment that surrounds the organization and exerts influence. Employee relations involve efforts to promote satisfaction and self-esteem of members within an organization. Attention to these relationships results in fair treatment, a healthy organizational climate, and long-term retention.

The structure of an organization is the sum of the relationships required to divide the work into a logical progression toward an objective. Structure dictates the relationships among people, work, and materials; and it involves power, responsibility, and division of labor. The external environment of an organization is part of a large social system. A single organization is only one among thousands that exist to influence each other. Society is the aggregate of all the external influences on organizations.

People compose the internal social system of an organization. They are attracted to an organization because it offers rewards that satisfy human needs. These rewards include promotion, security, recognition and, of course, pay. It is appropriate, then, to consider that organizations exist to serve people rather than to believe that people exist to serve organizations.

Recruiting the Right Candidate

Recruiting is the set of activities an organization uses to attract qualified candidates to help the organization achieve its objectives. Recruitment from the viewpoint of the employer is affected by several aspects; namely, the recruiting requirements set, the organization's policies, and the image of the employer in the community.

The Human Resources (HR) Department will request that managers specify the requirements considered ideal in applicants. The search for the right candidate must be realistic, and it begins with an examination of the specifications that are absolutely necessary for the job. These absolute basic specifications that each candidate is expected to meet serve as the beginning expectations for all recruits. Assuming all recruits begin the process of gaining employment on a level playing field, the most qualified applicants with the greatest likelihood for success in the job will emerge as finalists.

In most organizations, the HR Department's policies and practices may dictate who is recruited. Many organizations favor hiring from within. For practical purposes, this means that organizations only recruit from the outside for entry-level positions. This is a fair practice to reward loyal employees who are assured of a secure future and a chance at promotion. These organizations usually have strong training functions and encourage employees to develop new job skills. In technological positions where entry-level positions require educational preparation that occurs external to the organization, a steady stream of new recruits is very desirable, and recruitment activities centered around assuring a source of qualified candidates is another important function of human resource administration.

The company's image also affects recruitment. The image of a large employer generally held by the public can be the organization's most important drawing card. An organization's image is a complex situation; it is based largely on what the organization does and whether or not it is perceived as a good place to work. Healthcare organizations are lucky in this regard; most people view hospitals and clinics as a great service to the community. As a rule, healthcare professionals are highly regarded for the important work they do.

Sources of Recruits

Two sources of applicants are used by all employers; namely, internal (present employees) and external. As previously mentioned, promotion from within is strongly favored in today's workplace. An elaborate system of job posting to notify present employees of openings is commonplace. Another example of internal recruitment activities is when present employees are asked to encourage friends or relatives to apply. Employee referrals are a major recruiting source for employers. In a study of job-search behavior, one investigator reported that 31 percent of employees found their jobs through the help of family.

Media advertisements are another source of external recruits; the most common are newspaper help wanted ads. The other most effective method of print advertising for job applicants is professional journals. For large cities you will see billboards, subway and bus posters, radio, and television. A popular use of ad media is the telephone; nearly everyone reports experience with recorded want ad recordings.

Recruiters are used by many employers to secure candidates for top management positions and hard-to-find professionals. Professional recruiters have access to large pools of job hunters and can often match the qualifications of a candidate to a job very effectively. Most recruiters work directly with the employer to determine placement fees. The employer pays a premium for a job search conducted by a professional recruiter, but these "finding" fees are usually offset by the costs involved in conducting exhaustive searches without the assistance of head hunters.

Special events are another way that organizations secure recruits. Open houses, hosting receptions at professional meetings, making speeches at association meetings, local civic organizations, and area schools are all ways to attract attention to an employer. Most HR professionals report participation in job fairs as a major source of applicants. Job fairs appeal to job seekers who want to survey the employment opportunities in a particular area with a minimum of travel and interview expenses.

Effective Recruiting Strategies

- Create internship opportunities for students in area training programs. This allows the employer to provide trial run employment to determine if a student recruit is a potential future employee.
- Select recruiters that show interest in the applicant, that are enthusiastic about employment opportunities with the company, and that conduct a personal interview that is informative and nonstressful.
- Present a realistic view of the job to the candidate. A realistic job preview gives a person pertinent, truthful information about a job without distortion or exaggeration. Present the job as attractive, interesting, and stimulating in as balanced and truthful way possible.
- Maintain a working environment that promotes collaboration and consistency in policies and procedures. Establish clear lines of communication and encourage employees to problem solve and practice independently within their scope of practice.

Career Advancement Programming as an Aid to Retention

The development of a career advancement program requires multiple strategies by institutional or departmental management to enhance motivation, commitment, and effort of employees. Implementation of a well-developed program will be beneficial to patients, management, and employees by providing:

- Motivation for employees to commit to personal development.
- Improvement in versatility and flexibility that can improve and enhance employee scheduling and permit optimum employee utilization.

- Empowerment of employees through a system of equitable rewards to those who demonstrate professional attributes.
- Development of a recruitment incentive.
- Retention of employees through fulfillment that comes from personal professional development and advancement, as well as from exercise of expertise, judgment, and creativity.
- Improvement in the quality of patient care delivery through the increased knowledge and skills of the professionals serving them.
- Demonstration of a working partnership between management and employees with goals that improve and enhance patient care, increase workload efficiency and productivity and advance professional job satisfaction.*

Recruitment and retention advantages are high on the list of advantages cited by administrators interviewed on the subject of advancement programs. A Task Force on Career Strategies of the Summit on Manpower interviewed radiology managers in the summer of 1991 to determine the successes and advantages of career ladders and advancement strategies. Conclusions drawn from the survey results included the following real workplace advantages:

- Defined progression for advancement.
- Easier promotion.
- Mechanism for growth.
- More definitive pay grades.
- More responsibility given to first line supervisors.
- Opportunities for advancement of long-term employees.
- Market advantage for recruitment.
- Staff investment in department quality.
- Staff motivation.
- Improved flexibility of organizing work.

From the administrators' perspective, what worked best about their programs included:

- Employee buy-in of goals and objectives.
- More employee involvement.
- Objectivity in recognizing advancement.

---

* "Advancement Programs in the Workplace." Summit on Manpower. Sudbury, MA. May, 1992, p. 3.

- Cross-training in specialty areas.
- Increased staff flexibility.
- Decreased turnover.*

Administrators also reported positive results on employee satisfaction and productivity with advancement programs. Although the effects on productivity are difficult to measure, subjective assessments of worker's quality of work indicated that staff tried harder to achieve advancement levels. Satisfaction in the work environment was significantly noted by the Summit as:

- Increased job satisfaction.
- Improved morale and feedback.
- Eliminated employee turnover, except for better hours.
- Improved growth aspects.
- Increased positive attitudes.
- Improved professional attitude.

The radiologic professions have been stigmatized for years with the view that these kinds of jobs led nowhere. Technological development in the field from the mid-1960s has widened the horizons of opportunities for these occupations; mainly, job progression has taken the direction of technological specialization. The individual who desires to remain a radiographer stands to benefit greatly from this concept of career advancement programming.

Retention

Retaining good employees is a continual problem for healthcare managers. The obvious effects of this problem are brought to bear upon the quantity and quality of patient care. In the radiology department, a shortage of radiographers means that either the number of patients must be limited or the quality of work must be compromised. High turnover takes its toll on productivity, affects the morale of employees, and creates additional expenses for administration. Recruitment, orientation, pre-employment processing and the initial mistakes of new employees are additional turnover costs.

---

* "Advancement Programs in the Workplace." Summit on Manpower. Sudbury, MA. May 1992, p. 4.

High staff turnover usually indicates to management that problems exist within the structure of the organization. The primary
causes of turnover are related to problems associated with (1) the
employee, (2) work assignments, and (3) leadership.

Employee problems are often associated with the employee's
perception of the job or management's expectations of the individual's
performance. Employees may be inadequately prepared to assume
positions for which they are selected. These employee problems can
be minimized by carefully inducting individuals into the system. The
duties and responsibilities of a position should be described during
the initial interview. A thorough orientation program will also help
new employees assimilate new job responsibilities.

The work environment is another factor that contributes to turnover. Radiographers complain about the pressures of increasing
responsibility on the job, such as computerization, interventional
radiography techniques, and towering workloads. Another common complaint is that work assignments are too varied. When the
radiographer is continually assigned to different examination rooms
or to rotating shifts, or expected to perform special radiographic
examinations without proper in-service training, job dissatisfaction
is likely to surface.

The supervision an employee receives is also closely related to
turnover and job satisfaction. Employees expect their supervisors to
administer rewards when due, possess supervisory expertise, and
encourage group cohesiveness. The leadership of supervisors is
under constant scrutiny by the individuals they manage. Employees
cite lack of leadership and management skills, poor follow-through
on complaints, minimal interaction with the staff, and abuse of
authority as their major concerns about the leadership they receive
at work.

Aids to Retention

Radiology managers need to adopt administrative philosophies
that address the personal and professional growth of their employees. Radiologic professionals make a significant contribution to
patient care. The physicians who utilize their services and the admin-

istrators who coordinate radiology activities need to recognize the important work that is done.

The radiographer deserves professional recognition and a degree of autonomy at work. Autonomy could be accomplished by encouraging the decentralization of radiology departments into clinical sections. Doing this allows radiographers to manage their own work, to try new ideas, and to accept responsibility for the quality of radiography in their section. Decentralization within the radiology department also helps minimize the effects of the lack of opportunity for advancement except through administrative channels. Development of strong clinical responsibility by radiographers affords the opportunity for exceptional practitioners to gain specialist status and to be rewarded financially.

A formal retention program will depend on sound personnel practices and efforts to improve job satisfaction. The following management practices should be administered with retention as the objective:

1. Initial Interview. The applicant should be dealt with honestly. An unrealistic representation of the work environment and job content leads to disappointments and may result in early resignation.

2. Orientation. The new employee requires an induction to the organization that assures smooth assimilation into the work place. The employee should be informed of institutional expectations and standards of performance.

3. Communication. Good communication can be achieved through regular staff meetings and through individual interviews. Supervisors should encourage one-to-one encounters with employees that afford an exchange of concerns. When employees realize their input is welcome, needless frustration can be avoided.

4. Professional Development. The opportunity to participate in continuing education programs, workshops, and college courses should be offered to all personnel. Evidence of continuing education and increased competencies should form a basis for decisions made during performance appraisals and recommendations for promotion.

5. Salary and Benefits. Compensation should be commensurate with the level and experience of the employee. The salary and benefits plan of the institution should be competitive for its geographic location. A merit system for periodic salary adjustments has a positive impact on retention when coupled with a properly administered appraisal mechanism.

If job satisfaction is less than optimally achievable, the climate for a successful rate of retention is jeopardized. Abraham Maslow suggested that human needs are hierarchical, resulting in self-actualization. The satisfied employee, then, will prosper in an environment that provides interesting and challenging work, that allows self-expression, that assures recognition of a job well-done, and that encourages a feeling of accomplishment.

In 1989, the University of Michigan Medical Center adopted numerous expectations of management that focused on changing the workplace to one that recognized the talents of all people in the organization. There were 38 expectations of management; ten are related to retention:

1. Develop and support a work environment in which every employee's capability is improved.
2. Recognize that every employee wants to be a valued contributor and is capable of making an important contribution.
3. Select and promote people based on individual strengths, knowledge, leadership skills, and ability to work as part of a team.
4. Identify and compliment individuals on the area in which they perform well.
5. Identify, with employees, opportunities for their development.
6. Promote an environment of open communication.
7. Interact with employees on a regular basis.
8. Share appreciation of employees' contributions.
9. Create an atmosphere that promotes and encourages innovation and creativity.
10. Reward employees for participation and innovation through recognition, appreciation, and celebration.

What Do Workers Want From Their Jobs?

In talking about motives it is important to remember that people have many needs, all of which are continually competing for their behavior. No one person has exactly the same mixture or strength of these needs. There are some people who are driven mainly by money, others who are concerned primarily with security, and so on. While we must recognize individual differences, this does not mean that, as managers, we cannot make some predictions about which motives seem to be currently more prominent among our employees than others. According to Maslow, these are prepotent motives— those that are still *not* satisfied. An important question for managers to answer is, what do workers really want from their jobs?

Some interesting research has been conducted among employees in American industry in an attempt to answer this question. In one such study supervisors were asked to try to put themselves in a *worker's* shoes by ranking in order of importance a series of items that describe things workers may want from their jobs. It was emphasized that in ranking the items the supervisors should *not* think in terms of what they want but what they think a worker wants. In addition to the supervisors, the workers themselves were asked to rank these same items in terms of what *they* wanted most from their jobs. The results are given here (1 = highest and 10 = lowest in importance).

Figure 1.15 What Do Workers Want from Their Jobs?

	Supervisors	Workers
Good working conditions	4	9
Feeling "in" on things	10	2
Tactful disciplining	7	10
Full appreciation for work done	8	1
Management loyalty to workers	6	8
Good wages	1	5
Promotion and growth with company	3	7
Sympathetic understanding of personal problems	9	3
Job security	2	4
Interesting work	5	6

As is evident from the results, supervisors in this study generally ranked good wages, job security, promotion, and good working conditions as the things workers want most from their jobs. On the other hand, the workers felt that what they wanted most was full appreciation for work done, feeling "in" on things, and sympathetic understanding of personal problems—all incentives that seem to be related to affiliation and recognition motives. It is interesting to note that those things that workers indicated they wanted most from their jobs were rated by their foremen as least important. This study suggested very little sensitivity by supervisors as to what things were really most important to workers. Supervisors seemed to think that incentives directed to satisfy physiological and safety motives tended to be most important to their workers. Since these supervisors perceived their workers as having these motives, they acted, undoubtedly, as if these were their true motives. Therefore, these supervisors probably used the old reliable incentives—money, fringe benefits, and security—to motivate workers.*

1.11 PROMOTING YOUR OWN CAREER

Where do you start? First, understand that career planning is a very individualized process. Because you have a unique set of values, interests, skills, work and personal experiences, selling yourself to a perspective employer means understanding the requirements of various jobs and how your own characteristics match those jobs. Take some time to think about all of the following you/job related factors and form a picture in your mind about the kind of identity you will project in the job market.

- Do you understand the difference between having a "career" or just having "a job"?
- How do you feel about status and prestige in a job?
- What do the financial rewards need to be to attract you?
- Do you care where the job is?
- Are you looking for a large or small company?
- What are your strengths and weaknesses? List them.

---

*Hersey, P. and Blanchard, K. Management of Organizational Behavior. Englewood Cliffs, N.J., Prentice-Hall, Inc. 1982, pp. 41, 42.

- What kind of work most interests you?
- Are you trained to perform the work you are seeking?
- What special skills and education do you have?

Many first-time job hunters and also those who have been out of the job-seeking mode for a long time will accept the help of professional career counselors. Vocational testing is often helpful in verifying one's self-analysis of job interests, and it can also reveal hidden personal characteristics that could lead to other unexpected career opportunities. Once you understand your own personality and intellectual abilities, planning a job search is the next step.

The Job Search

As a radiologic professional you will face a number of possible employers. Because you possess specific skills that are sought by healthcare providers everywhere, looking for job openings should be a pleasant exercise. But how do you narrow the available job opportunities and where do you look for job possibilities? Newspapers and professional journals are the two major sources of job openings. The classified ads, especially in the Sunday edition of all major newspapers, will provide a lot of job information. Also, talk to family, friends, teachers, and other professional contacts that may know of job leads. When you discover a potential position, then consider these important questions about the employment place that you are considering:

- Is there an opening for someone with your skills, aptitude, and goals?
- Is there advancement opportunity?
- What kind of record does the company have for promoting within?
- Are there professional development programs?
- Is it a pleasant environment in which to work?
- Is the company financially sound?

Resume Rules

A resume is a clearly written snapshot of who you are, what you have accomplished, and where you would like to be next. Many candidates with apparently the same credentials apply for the same job, but most are eliminated during an initial screening of resumes. This happens when you don't look good on paper. Conveying to a prospective employer that you have the credentials, experience, and ability to do a good job requires that you present that information effectively. Your resume is an advertisement, a tool you use to market yourself. Effectively advertising yourself means highlighting your best qualities while de-emphasizing your deficiencies.

To make a positive impression, a resume needs to look good, be well organized, and be complete. The most popular form of resume presentation is the chronological method. In this form, work experience is reported in reverse chronological order. The most recent (current) job is described first (it is thought that you are only as good as your last act). Therefore, the bulk of your resume should dwell on all your very recent accomplishments. If you have performed many jobs in one place with progressively greater responsibility in each, be sure to show that career growth and ability to take on increased duties.

The chronological resume can be up to four pages in length, and it is written in a confident and persuasive style aimed towards one objective: getting the interview.

Elements of a chronological resume will include:

- Name, address, telephone.
- Summary of experience.
- Career objective.
- Education.
- Experience.
- Military service, if any.
- Professional affiliations.
- Personal interests.
- Personal data.

The resume must be neat and accurate, and free of typos, misspelled words, or grammatical errors. It should be submitted with a cover letter that introduces the applicant to the employer. The letter is only a quick introduction and should not repeat the information found in the resume. A well-prepared resume will enhance the opportunity for an interview, and it's that interview that will lead you to be the candidate of choice (see Figure 1.16, sample resume).

Figure 1.16 Sample Chronological Resume

Charles L. Thompson
3986 Creekside Circle
New Bedford, MA 02740

(508) 586-4726 (H)   (508) 661-3870 (W)

Summary	Experienced hospital manager with a successful record of achievement in radiology department administration.
Objective	A challenging position in radiology management, utilizing analytical and problem solving activities.

Education

September, 1980–
May, 1984

University of South Carolina
School of Health Related Professions
Major—Radiological Administration
Bachelor of Science

September, 1976–
May, 1980

Hillcrest High School
Major —Business Administration
Diploma

Experience

May, 1988–Present

Radiological Administrator, HCA
Mary Coker Hospital, Longbridge, CT
Responsibilities included the coordination and daily supervision of imaging services in a 265 bed general community hospital. With an operating budget of $1.6 million, the department performed 91,000 total procedures per year with 23 FTEs.

May, 1984–May, 1988

Technical Director, Summer Bend
Community Hospital, Plymouth, MA
Responsible for all technical aspects of a busy radiology department in a 175 bed general community hospital. Also functioned part-time as a special procedures technologist when needed and conducted all quality control monitoring in the department.

Affiliations

1985 American Healthcare Radiology Administrators
1988 Connecticut Society of Radiologic Technologists
1989 Longbridge JAYCEES

Personal Interests

Various fund raising projects associated with the local JAYCEE chapter, hunting, fishing and golf.

Personal Data

Married, Methodist, 5/1/61 date of birth

The Employment Interview

You must perform well at the employment interview to get the job. Prepare for that interview carefully; you should dress according to the appearance codes that exist in the place you wish to work. An important aspect of your interview will be how well you might fit into the existing organization; therefore, try to look the part. Do some homework on the place. Find out:

- Where it is located.
- Who runs the organization.
- What they do best.
- If they are financially sound.
- Who is the competition.
- How they are organized.
- What their plans are for future growth.

Consider getting an interview as a major accomplishment. It means that you are a competitor and that speaks well of your resume preparation, networking skills, and experience up to this point. The employment interview will be a challenge that you can meet and do very well because you are interested in succeeding.

The actual interview is a conversation with a purpose. The purpose is to discover whether you are the right person for the job. The only way the interviewer can determine if you are a possible match is to ask questions. Your answers need to be quick, informed, and honest. To assure the best answers to a series of rapid fire probing questions, you need to be prepared. Some typical interview questions are listed below:

- Why do you want to work here?
- What kind of career have you planned for yourself?
- How did you prepare for that career choice?
- What are you looking for in an employer?
- Can you relate previous experience to this job?
- What are your strengths and weaknesses?
- How did you choose the schools you attended?
- What has been your greatest achievement?
- Can you describe your management style?

- Are you a leader?
- How do you plan to continue to grow professionally?

How to Interview Your Future Boss*

At a job interview you're mostly concerned about how you come across to your potential employer.

You should be equally interested in how that person comes across to you, says employment consultant Jeffrey Mayer.

Pay close attention to your gut reactions during your conversation regarding:

- How she asks you questions.
- How she listens when you speak.
- How she responds to your questions and comments.

In fact, Mayer suggests that you interview your prospective boss! Ask about his career:

- How long has he been with the firm?
- What positions has he previously held?
- Where has he worked?

(In the back of your mind ask yourself, "Is he on the move? Will he be here in the next few years? How would a change in his position affect my career?")

Ask about her management style:

- What forms of office communication does she prefer (regular staff meetings, impromptu meetings, memos)?
- How available will she be to answer your questions?
- How much time will be spent training you?
- What will be expected of you as a new employee (e.g. will you be expected to be at your desk 8:00 to 5:00, to work weekends, to set your own hours)?

Look around at his office: is it well-organized or does his desk look like a toxic waste dump? Do there seem to be a lot of unfinished work

*Jeffrey J. Mayer, *Find the Job You've Always Wanted in Half the Time and With Half the Effort*, (1992), Contemporary Books, 180 North Michigan Ave., Chicago, IL 60601. As adapted by the Pryor Report Vol 9 (1):9, 1993.

projects and unanswered phone messages lying around? (This means you may be stuck handling crises stemming from lost material and overdue tasks.)

How considerate was the interviewer of your time? Were there interruptions as you talked? Did she take notes?

Before the interview ends, says Mayer, ask two questions:

1. What else can I tell you about myself or my career experience that we haven't discussed?
2. What is your assessment of this interview?

These questions will help clear up any misunderstandings and let you know where you stand.

The interview is your window of opportunity to employment; therefore, it is important to be impressive at the interview by being well prepared. It is also important that they remember you. A short thank you letter after the interview is an effective means of communicating your thanks and continued interest in an employment opportunity with that employer.

1.12 CUSTOMER RELATIONS
Creating a Consumer Oriented Workforce

The business of providing healthcare services is dependent upon an increasing trend of patients playing prominent roles in selecting their own healthcare provider. This tough new challenge is being met with strategies for improving patient relations and for enhancing the hospital environment. These, along with educating the community about specialized hospital services, are topics being examined in virtually all facilities that are seeking that competitive edge. It is essential that the environment be one where caring attitudes prevail and where care givers get caught up in the spirit of hospitality.

This "high-touch" approach to humanizing a high-tech environment is a client-centered philosophy that appreciates the needs and expectations of patients and that sets in place a process that promotes excellent patient relations and consumer satisfaction.

There will always be a tremendous diversity of people on a hospital staff; but when one asks patients about their favorite employee, the responses are mostly the same: everyone likes to be around persons who are responsive, know how to listen, seem to care, have a sense of humor, show respect, and display warmth.

How to create a more consumer-oriented work force that will help healthcare organizations compete successfully in a competitive market is a current principal focus of human resources management. Employees are a visible and integral component of marketing strategy. With all this attention on growing competitive pressures, it is not surprising that top management is asking for quality recruits and is placing more emphasis on training persons who show an aptitude for the desired behaviors of customer relations.

The Process Begins with Selection

This customer relations focus changes the process of employee selection and dictates that screening procedures are set up that provide for the applicants with the greatest potential for successful public contact to be identified quickly.

This means that customer relations skills need to be included in specifications and that the employment interview be structured so that some assessment can be made of the interviewee's skill in handling difficult situations.

A formal retention program should be administered with employee satisfaction as the primary objective and consumer satisfaction as the primary result of that satisfaction. An applicant should receive a realistic representation of the work environment and the importance of good public contact skills as specific job content. The new employee should be inducted into the organization smoothly and should understand the institutional expectations and standards of performance. Good communication is achieved by supervisors encouraging one-to-one encounters that emphasize human relations skills, and supervisors should model the behavior that is expected during encounters.

Customer Relations in the Performance Appraisal Process

The performance appraisal process should reflect an evaluation of the dimension of customer relations. A measurement of human interaction has been historically present in most performance appraisal systems. This elusive standard has been measured globally at best, and it misses the mark when specific behaviors related to attitudes and actions that promote favorable customer relations are desired. The performance-based appraisal system must include specific references to customer relations that attend to appropriate demeanor manifested by: courtesy, friendliness, concern, sensitivity, cooperation, and respect.

The performance appraisal system will reinforce the values that the organization holds important. The reinforcement of desired behaviors, with an appraisal system that offers positive and negative consequences for action, is essential to support any theme in an enterprise. When the appraisal process is initiated, it is important to emphasize that customer relations ranks up there with the other prerequisite skills for performing work.

Consumerism as a Marketing Strategy

Orientation to customer relations expectations should carry an implicit message that an alternative, cohesive, productive, and motivated staff with a clear understanding of what is required to satisfy the public is the desired end result. All employees, regardless of their roles in the organization, should understand that they have the responsibility for determining the future. Every employee and every department is needed to maximize patient and physician satisfaction. This customer relations aspect of marketing is an important strategy for keeping current business and encouraging more. This marketing strategy looks at the patient, both as someone in need of healthcare and as someone with real purchasing power.

The organization's expectations for customer satisfaction must be clear from the onset. The customer relations training should translate marketing concerns into practical demonstrations of how relations skills build satisfaction and promote wellness for patients. Brief courteous encounters have a significant affect on setting the tone for a patient's experiences in the healthcare environment. Total involvement of all staff members in courtesy awareness assures a general enabling atmosphere. Special emphasis on complaint resolution with particular attention for dealing with complaints with competence and compassion is another important objective of consumer satisfaction skill development.

Summary

- Train your employees so that they are certified ready to meet the public.
- Know who deals with the public in your organization and see that they continue to meet the high standards you have set.
- Be aware of how much public contact should be expected of an employee and avoid overloading someone with too much high pressure interaction.
- Pay attention to those who are doing the job right and give them recognition.

1.13 CUSTOMER RELATIONS TRAINING
A Request for Proposal Example

Understanding and succeeding in the hospital business means that prosperous healthcare enterprises have identified their customers and have positioned their institutions for the competitive edge. The hospital as a business has evolved into a complex organization that utilizes elements of public relations, marketing, and customer relations to assure its position in the marketplace.

The issue of "hospital hospitality" has become a topic that is being examined in virtually all facilities that are seeking that competitive edge. A heightened awareness of the importance of delivering better service in an enthusiastic manner are key goals to a proposed program. Finding the vendor that suits the unique environment of your hospital is a task for which the Request for Proposal (RFP) to provide customer relations training is designed. **An example of this RFP format follows.**

Introduction

It is the intention of the hospital to solicit proposals for conducting a customer relations program for its employees.

The hospital seeks a high-touch approach to humanizing its high-tech environment. That is, a customer-centered philosophy that assesses the needs and expectations of patients, and a process set in place that promotes and evaluates the practice of customer relations and consumer satisfaction. The objective of the project is to train all employees in the techniques of customer relations.

Background

A general description of the hospital (size, locale, and scope of services) would be needed to introduce the perspective vendor to the organization.

Scope of Work

The contractor shall design and conduct a customer relations program for all hospital employees. The program should focus on raising employees' consciousness and enhancing their caring attitude in order to create a warmer and more caring environment for all types of hospital guests, patients, visitors, physicians, and other employees.

The program should identify problem areas, design effective mechanisms for developing interpersonal skills and behavioral standards, and develop appropriate evaluation techniques to measure the success of the program and enhance its continuing effectiveness over a two-year period.

The hospital expects the customer relations program to achieve the following objectives:

A. Raise awareness of the personal value each employee brings to their job.
B. Help employees recognize their impact on the work environment and hospital image.
C. Teach polite, efficient, and supportive forms of communication.
D. Provide the skills that staff members require to defuse emotionally charged situations.
E. Build a solid reputation for quality customer relations and patient satisfaction that will attract patients and top physicians.

F. Help staff members develop a clear picture of the need to improve patient satisfaction and the staff member's role in attaining higher levels of patient satisfaction.
G. Help staff members perceive patients as consumers who are selecting medical services.

The contractor shall provide all personnel, equipment, and expertise to design and conduct a customer relations program utilizing the "train-the-trainer" approach. The number of trainers from the facility should be adequate to provide the training of all employees in a reasonable time frame. The contractor will participate in the selection of the trainers during on-site interviews. A post evaluation of the effectiveness of customer relations efforts will be designed by the contractor. A plan for the continuation of customer relations training will be designed by the contractor after the initial hospital employees have matriculated through the program.

Organizational and Management Plan

1. An explanation of the manner in which the offerer plans to ensure completion and delivery of high quality services within the proposed time constraints.
2. Identity of the individuals who will work on the project together with their level of involvement.

Experience and Qualifications

1. Offerers should provide a list of reference institutions where similar customer relations programs have been conducted. The list should include the name of a contact person and telephone number. The hospital reserves the right to contact referenced institutions.
2. Resumes of key individuals assigned to the project should be included.
3. Offerers should specify the method and regularity of expected contact with the hospital staff.

Project Budget

1. Offerers should include a line item budget including all cost categories.

Award Criteria

Proposals will be evaluated by a review panel on the basis of the following criteria that are listed in order of importance (see Figure 1.17).

A. Technical Approach—the quality of offerer's overall approach to performing the tasks set forth in the Scope of Work.
B. Offerer's Qualifications—the offerer's qualifications and experience in conducting customer relations training, particularly in a healthcare institution.
C. Understanding the Environment—an understanding of the environment of the hospital and knowledge of training employees in a healthcare setting.
D. Cost.
E. Project staffing and organization including references.

Figure 1.17

**Evaluation Instrument
Request for Proposal
Customer Relations**

Name of Offerer (vendor):_____

Name of Evaluator:_____

1. **TECHNICAL APPROACH**–The overall approach to fulfill the work as set forth in the Scope and Objectives of the Proposal (MAXIMUM 30 POINTS)

2. **OFFERER'S QUALIFICATIONS**–Including references and past performance qualifications and experience in conducting customer relations training, particularly in a healthcare institution (MAXIMUM 25 POINTS)

3. **UNDERSTANDING THE ENVIRONMENT**–Offerer should demonstrate an understanding of the environment of the hospital and knowledge of training employees in a healthcare setting. (MAXIMUM 20 POINTS)

4. **COST**–Offerer should provide a breakdown of costs, including estimated travel expenses and method of payments. (MAXIMUM 15 POINTS)

5. **PROJECT**–Staffing and organization (MAXIMUM 10 POINTS)

Grand Total: (Maximum 100 points)

NOTE: Comments should be made on separate sheet of paper attached to this evaluation.

Appendix A

SUGGESTED CRITERIA FOR SELECTING A CONTRACT SERVICE PROVIDER

- How long has the contractor been in business?
- What experience has the contractor had in providing services to facilities similar to yours?
- Will the contractor guarantee the quality of the service to be provided?
- How familiar is the contractor with your facility, your service area and your customers?
- Does the contractor have the resources and capability to provide the services you require?
- Will the contractor provide the management expertise and professional image you want and need?
- Does the contractor understand how you provided service in the past and how it is currently being provided?
- Does the contractor understand your goals and objectives?
- Will the contractor assist you in meeting regulatory agency requirements?
- Will the contract service reduce the administrative time you now spend on providing the service?
- What is the general appearance and readability of the contractor's proposal?
- Is the contractor offering you a customized program, designed specifically to meet your needs?
- Did the contractor address all of your issues and concerns?
- How comfortable are you with the contractor's approach?
- How did the contractor demonstrate desire for your business?
- Did the contractor make it clear which individual(s) would be directly responsible for providing the contracted service?
- What did you like best about the contractor and what did you like least?
- Were the contractor's references favorable? Who, beyond the references provided, did you contact?

1.14 COMMUNICATING WITH MEDICAL STAFF

The Key to Success

What is the common denominator of successful healthcare facilities today? Is it service delivered in a cheerful and efficient manner, the latest in technological instrumentation, an expert and innovative administration? Each of these denominators are important but none equals the necessity of great physician relations. Here exists an irreplaceable healthcare basic tenet; physicians are essential to patient care.

Today as always, physicians are held in high esteem; hospitals cater to their needs, and administration is involving medical staff in many major decisions. The most valued members of medical staffs are those who emerge with the qualities of business savvy, expert medical knowledge, and patient understanding. Smart hospital administrators are pursuing the concept of physician relations by opening departments that cater to special physician needs. Guest relations programs in hospitals are placing a premier emphasis on physician relationships, which is a logical order of attention because it is the physician who is responsible for the patients and visitors found in the hospital. Successful healthcare facilities recognize the *physician* as a principal guest.

Strategies for Improved Relations

The thrust of doctor-focused communications should demonstrate mutual benefits to the physician and to the hospital. One strategy, the development of an office of physician relations, is a relationship management strategy that centralizes physician services into a line function. A physician liaison officer is an ombudsman and acts as a facilitator to promote and resolve physician concerns. The strength of this strategy is demonstrated by physician acceptance of the sincerity of the hospital's efforts to monitor physician complaints and resolve problems.

Physician recruitment programs targeted at assisting new physicians to establish practices are usually mutually beneficial arrangements. Physician recruitment programs are especially useful when seeding efforts are targeted to clinical areas, where the hospital desires to increase admissions. In addition, assisting high admitting loyal physicians in expanding their practices will always positively impact the size of a hospital's admissions.

Expanding the referral base of tertiary care centers through geographic outreach will also significantly impact physician relations. These programs concentrate on building ties between rural primary care physicians and tertiary specialists. Outreach usually results in measurable increases in geographic market share and admissions.

A very useful communications device is personal contact. Relationships with physicians, as in the community and other healthcare organizations, are important benchmarks of marketing effectiveness. Hospitals and physician specialists are dependent upon the excellent relationships that feed referrals. There are four critical functions being attempted by hospital sales forces. They are: service development, attitude management, education, and relationship building. These critical functions translate into marketing concepts. To implement marketing concepts, competent marketing manpower is required. Hospitals that have established an aggressive, targeted sales force to increase hospital utilization report amazing success in incremental services directly accounted to sales activity.

Physician Bonding Approaches

A shortcut from the systematic staff building that has been described thus far is the practice of attracting and creating superstars. When an established expert specialist in a profitable clinical area can be recruited to further build a reputation and major program, years of development time can be saved. The outstanding reputation of one physician can attract significant business to their specialty and related areas. Recruiting a superstar requires a major investment on the part of the hospital. This investment is at risk if a competitor is able to lure that superstar away.

Computer networks have the potential for hospitals to influence the critical links in its referral network. When a computer connects primary care physicians and specialists with the hospital, scheduling patient appointments, receiving test results, financial information, and medical records are readily available to the physician's office personnel.

Some commonly agreed on ways to strengthen hospital-physician relations include the following:

- Encourage interaction and relationship building between the board, medical staff, and management by putting physicians on committee boards.
- Involve physicians in decision making. Target younger physicians for earlier and more aggressive participation on committees. The more directly they are involved in hospital committee work the better they'll understand the business of the hospital and the more closely aligned they'll become.
- Assess managed care and what is happening in the community. Consider presenting educational programs to bring physicians up to speed in terms of what managed care is all about and how they can use it proactively as an opportunity.
- Offer physician practice support. Consider presenting a package that involves a turnkey operation that provides billing, office staff, and equipment for items that are required to get the practice up and running from day one. By contributing management expertise, the hospital can control revenues, provide practice continuity, establish affirmed successions, and retain its identity.
- Play a role as a catalyst in bringing practices together and supporting merger and acquisition discussions. This type of involvement can build stronger loyalties to an institution.
- Place a senior staff member in attendance at all of the medical staff committee meetings and department meetings to immediately address issues raised by physicians.*

Summary

In the current atmosphere of competition and of changes in technology and utilization, administrators who don't recognize the imperative of fine physician relations may find a gradual erosion of their admissions basis. Administrators cannot ignore the fact that physicians are customers with the ultimate power to make or break

---

*Berger, S. and Sudman, S.K. Physician/Hospital Trends for the 1990s Raise Some Red Flags. *Healthcare Executive* MAR/APRIL, 1992, p. 15.

a hospital. With reimbursement shrinking, administrators need to secure and expand patient volume to maintain desired levels of revenue.

Keep in mind that a mission of effectiveness in physician relations will include the management of many needs that will meaningfully engage physicians as team members. Physicians will seek affiliations with facilities that offer the technological advantage because the consumer assumes competence through those linkages. This technological advantage requires that hospital administration assume a constant posture of technology assessment.

Physicians also compete among themselves so they will look to be associated with those who stress the service component of medical care. Consumers are largely unable to evaluate medical competence. Consumers select and evaluate their doctors based on service criteria, and this evaluation is greatly determined by the hospital environment that they encounter.

Finally, healthcare is in a liability crisis, and there is a predisposition for litigation. Physicians cannot afford malpractice suits because they are expensive and ruin reputations. For that reason physicians have a stake in strong working relationships with hospital staff. They depend on the hospital to assure a safe environment for patient care.

Everyone stands to gain from improved physician relations. A meaningful strategy builds on the potential mutual benefits of all involved; namely, the patient who is cared for, the physician practice that is enhanced, and the hospital that survives.

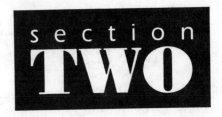

TECHNOLOGY

2.1 RADIOLOGY INFORMATION SYSTEMS

Radiology Information Systems (RIS) have been around since the early 1970s. As the 1990s begin, approximately 1,000 RISs are installed in U. S. hospitals, thus leaving another 6,000 hospitals, clinics, and imaging centers without this efficiency improving technology. There are many RIS vendors; at least fifty U.S. software vendors vie for their share of a wide open market.

Radiology departments seem to get passed over as candidates for information systems in favor of other departments; namely, the laboratory (2,500 systems installed as of 1990). RIS adoption has been slow in radiology. Radiology departments have taken longer to automate than labs and pharmacies despite the fact that the computer management applications were recognized by radiology early in the 1970s.

In recent years, capital expenditures in radiology have been made in new technology, magnetic-resonance imagers, PET scanners, and more CT. Computerization in imaging is evolving in three distinct tracks: x-ray has gone "digital" with MRI and CT, radiology information systems are now emerging in importance, and the future holds the use of picture archiving systems (PACS).

RIS development is spurred by three interrelated factors. First, advanced technologies such as MRI, PET, CT, and SPECT increase the acceptance of computer information processing. All of these modalities, when added to the menu of radiological examinations already available, mean more exam volume. A real critical need for automated office functions has become apparent to most busy departments. Second, the cost of new technology in radiology has tripled in the last decade. Collecting the data necessary to build proformas to support the acquisition of new technology is made so much easier with an RIS. Third, the prospective payment system has really put a squeeze on the perennially profitable radiology department. Radiology must become more efficient to survive the economic scrutiny of today's healthcare environment. Radiology is no longer the "cash cow" of the past.

The Need for Efficient Information Management

The complexity of radiology management today calls for computerized solutions. Radiology Information Systems are the most valuable management tool available today to assist in the recording and analysis of the myriad of information collected for patient care in imaging. If the question of how to accomplish increased efficiency with the shortest length of payback is raised, then the answer is RIS. Computer-based information systems automate the basic functions that occur in the department every day.

There are two major components to all RIS systems: the hardware and the software. The hardware for an RIS consists of the computer, storage devices, terminals, printers, cables, and input devices (such as bar code readers). The RIS may be part of an integrated system, where the mainframe is located elsewhere, or an independent system found in the radiology department. The software in an RIS organizes the information collected into a useable form. The software dictates the functions of the system. Commonly performed functions of nearly all radiology information systems available today include:

- Patient information.
- Scheduling (Order entry).
- Patient tracking.
- Inventory control.
- Charge capture.
- Report generation.
- Bar code reading.
- Report inquiry.
- Report printing.
- Film file management.
- Teaching file management.
- Management reporting.

Selecting the RIS

Preparation is the key to selecting a radiology information system. The activities that take place before the search begins lay the foundation for a successful purchase. Preliminary tasks include:

- Putting together a dedicated committee.
- Developing a shared vision.
- Analyzing the current manual system.
- Setting expectations for the RIS.
- Planning for selecting the system.

The selection committee should include representatives from all parts of the hospital affected by the RIS. Including representatives from all applicable areas of the hospital gives the committee the collected wisdom and different viewpoints necessary to do a critical review of available systems. Ideally, the chairman of the RIS search committee should be from the radiology department. This person should be thoroughly familiar with the flow of information in the department and have knowledge of daily operations. It is helpful from the onset if the radiology representative is slated to be the eventual system manager. Thus, this person invests his or her energy in a personal future and has added motivation to conduct the best search possible. Do not underestimate the effort it takes to choose a system. For example, the search process may involve travel for site visits, factory tours, and a substantial time commitment. A search for an RIS can take up to a year to complete; therefore, each member of the committee needs to be willing to dedicate the necessary time, energy, and expertise to the project.

A shared vision gives the committee a sense of purpose and provides direction for thinking. A shared vision motivates an entire committee with a view of the future, an opportunity for imagination, a chance to plan ahead and a charge to integrate the RIS acquisition into the organization's overall goals and mission statement. Members of the committee should spend time discussing why the hospital is buying an RIS. Because the purchase will affect the hospital's future, the committee needs to understand how the RIS will fit into the long-term mission. A shared vision seeks to examine where the hospital will expand and grow, what healthcare will be like ten years ahead, and if the RIS will really improve the delivery of patient care.

Before considering an RIS, look critically at the current manual system and identify its strengths and weaknesses. An RIS does more than just replace an existing paper system; it will bring about many positive changes. A successful RIS installation will streamline and improve present procedures.

Setting expectations for the RIS that will fit into the hospital's overall mission for information management is a major function of the selection committee. RISs can provide solutions to productivity problems, reduce employee expenses, aid in continuous quality improvement activities, and improve overall patient services. If one of the hospital's goals is to provide the best radiological care possible to its patients, the technologists and other radiology employees must be freed of tedious paperwork.

Planning for selection is the final preliminary task of RIS evaluation. A decision-making mechanism needs to be in place to guide the committee towards eventual selection of a system. A list of questions and a standard form to keep the information organized will be a valuable evaluation tool. The form should allow for objective and subjective assessments of the systems under evaluation. A more formal decision analysis technique will involve weighted scales. The committee must have in place a plan for making a final decision before the time arrives to make the all important choice.

Questions to Consider When Planning an RIS Evaluation

1. Does your committee include members from areas of the hospital affected by the system?
2. Does the committee include users?
3. Are committee members committed to the task?
4. Is the committee the right size?
5. Is there understanding of the hospital's overall mission?
6. Will the RIS fit in the mission statement?
7. Has enough brainstorming occurred about the future system?
8. Has the paper-based system been fully analyzed?
9. How will the RIS improve current procedures?
10. Will the RIS eliminate old problems?
11. How will the RIS improve productivity? Are these productivity improvements measurable?

Evaluating Radiology Information Systems

Before the decision is made to buy, the committee will evaluate RISs from many different perspectives. The committee will look at a range of issues besides cost. Those issues include areas to evaluate such as the following:

- Overall system performance such as speed, reliability, and safety from data loss.
- System features such as user friendliness, configurable vs. programmable, security, reporting capabilities, and access to data.
- Hardware features such as workstations and connectivity.
- Additional expenses such as training, site preparation, system configuration and programming, software upgrades, foreign system interfaces, mounting devices, and new input devices.

Questions to Consider During Evaluation

1. Does the RIS provide the functions the department needs?
2. Do the RIS applications closely match the current manual system?
3. Will applications planned for the future be useful to your department?
4. Is the system fast enough?
5. Will the system still respond quickly when many people are using it?
6. What safeguards are built in to prevent system failure?
7. Is the system easy to use?
8. Are there "help functions" to aid the inexperienced user?
9. Are screens designed in a logical order, easy to read, and comfortable with which to work?
10. How easy is it to make program changes?
11. What parts of the system are reconfigurable?
12. What happens to information already in storage after system reconfiguration or reprogramming?
13. Is vendor support for problems available locally? By telephone?

14. What are the security features of the system?
15. Can you configure your own reports?
16. Will database access compromise daily functions?
17. Will the hardware provide enough processing power for future applications?
18. Does the system have connectivity?
19. What will the system cost to maintain?
20. Is the vendor financially stable and able to maintain and develop the system over the long term?

Implementing the RIS in Your Department

Look for a vendor that offers a comprehensive implementation plan, a quality training program, a program of planned maintenance, and a commitment of long-term support. Installing a new computer system is no easy task; a smooth installation will depend on the vendor's preparation. A solid implementation plan will consist of site planning, hardware placement, inservice training, and support. Committee members should use the opportunity of site visits to inquire how well installations went in other hospitals. The major steps in an RIS installation that when executed successfully will assure a smooth implementation are:

- Write a detailed implementation plan.
- Identify the implementation team.
- Prepare the site.
- Train the implementation team.
- Determine all interfaces.
- Define displays and reports.
- Develop operating procedures.
- Develop teaching tools for users.
- Install and test hardware.
- Install and check software.
- Connect all interfaces.
- Test the system.
- Monitor the conversion.
- Train the users.

Questions to Consider About Implementation

1. What kind of an implementation plan will the vendor supply?
2. How long will the installation take?
3. Is the system easy to use?
4. What kind of training will the vendor provide?
5. What kind of support for hardware and software exists? Is it vendor supplied?
6. How are system upgrades installed?
7. Is service local?
8. Does the vendor offer support training to hospital personnel?
9. What percentage "uptime" does the vendor report in their installed base?
10. Will the system require a fulltime manager?

Radiology Information Systems Are for Now and the Future

Radiology managers are finding numerous reasons to support and to justify the acquisition of RISs. Reduced patient stays may be attributed to more time-effective scheduling of exams, patient and physician complaints are reduced because operations are streamlined; productivity analysis is made easy, thus justifying existing and future personnel; and increased efficiencies allow more exams to be conducted by fewer personnel. Nearly all managers report significant lost charges recaptured, which speeds payback on the RIS investment. Another great benefit of an RIS is that it allows radiology professionals to concentrate on patient service rather than on good paperwork.

The "blue sky" plan for RIS is interfacing digital imaging techniques with information systems to create filmless, paperless radiology departments. Picture Archival Communication Systems (PACS) now currently available will store images on optical discs and display the images on high resolution video viewers. Putting RIS and PACS together will be the radiology department of the future. The American College of Radiology and the National Electronics Manufacturers Association are working together to set standards for imaging equipment and computers. These NEMA-ACR standards will insure that future integration of tests, graphics, and images can more easily occur in the future.

Appendix A—Major RIS Vendors

ADAC Laboratories
540 Alder Drive
Milpitas, CA 95030
(800) 538-8531

The Compucare Co.
12110 Sunset Hills Rd., #500
Reston, VA 22090
(703) 709-2426

BDM Information Systems Ltd.
15 Innovation Blvd., 4th Fl.
Saskatoon, SK Canada S7N 2X8
(306) 933-3000

Dalcon Computer Systems
1321 Murfreesboro Road
Nashville, TN 37217
(615) 366-4300

CHC Inc.
5 Greenway Plaza, #1900
Houston, TX 77046
(800) CHC-INFO

Dimensional Medicine Inc.
10901 Bren Road East
Minnetonka, MN 55343
(612) 938-8280

CPSI
6600 Wall Street
Mobile, AL 36695
(205) 639-8100

Datacare Inc.
1000 N. Ashley Drive, #800
Tampa, FL 33602
(813) 221-3077 ext. 2151

Cerner Corporation
2800 Rockcreek Parkway
Kansas City, MO 64117
(816) 221-1024

E.I. du Pont de Nemours & Co.,
Med. Products—Diag. Imaging
2 Northpoint Drive, #200
Houston, TX 77060
(713) 878-6400

First Coast Systems Inc.
6430 Southpoint Pkwy, #250
Jacksonville, FL 32216
(904) 296-4200

First Data Corp.,
Health Systems Group
10101 Claude Freeman Dr.
Charlotte, NC 28262
(704) 549-7000

Gerber Alley
6575 The Corners Pkwy.
Norcross, GA 30092
(404) 441-7793

GTE Health Systems
175 S. West Temple
Salt Lake City, UT 84101
(801) 539-4900

HBO & Co.
301 Perimeter Center North
Atlanta, GA 30346
(404) 393-6000

Health Data Sciences Corp.
268 W. Hospitality Lane
San Bernardino, CA 92408
(714) 888-3282

HealthVISION America Corp.
300 Queen Anne Ave. North, #505
Seattle, WA 98109
(206) 624-0219

Hospital Computer Systems
Monmouth Shores Corp.
Park, P.O. Box 2430
Farmingdale, NJ 07727
(908) 938-5600

IBAX Healthcare Systems
587 E. Sanlando Springs Dr.
Longwood, FL 32750
(407) 831-8444 ext. 2980

IDX Systems Corp.
1400 Shelburne Road
Burlington, VT 05402
(802) 862-1022

Lanier Worldwide Inc.
Voice Products Division
1700 Chantilly Dr., N.E.
Atlanta, GA 30324
(800) 648-6423

Management Systems
Associates Inc.
5580 Centerview Drive
Raleigh, NC 27606
(919) 851-6177

Medical Information Technology
Inc. (MEDITECH)
Meditech Circle
Westwood, MA 02090
(617) 821-3000

Megasource Inc.
2600 S. Telegraph Rd., #200
Bloomfield Hills, MI 48302
(313) 332-9403

National Medical Computer
Services
8928 Terman Court
San Diego, CA 92121
(619) 566-5800 ext. 479

PHAMIS Inc.
401 2nd Ave. South, #200
Seattle, WA 98104
(206) 689-1328

Professional Medical
Management Inc.
7671 Silverthorn, S.E.
Ada, MI 49301
(616) 243-2130

RADMAN Inc.
2811 Wilshire Blvd., #690
Santa Monica, CA 90403
(310) 828-3600

SMS Inc.
51 Valley Stream Parkway
Malvern, PA 19317
(215) 219-6300

Shebele Inc.
14 Tenby Road
Havertown, PA 19083
(800) 795-2329

Siemens Medical Systems
186 Wood Ave. South
Iselin, NJ 08830
(908) 321-4564

Sunquest Information Systems
4801 E. Broadway
Tucson, AZ 85711
(602) 570-2000

Swearingen Software Inc.
10235 West Little York, #418
Houston, TX 77040
(800) 992-1767

TDS Healthcare Systems
200 Ashford Center N.
Atlanta, GA 30338
(404) 847-5304

3M Health Information Systems
575 West Murray Boulevard
Murray, UT 84157-0900
(800) 367-2447

Weichinger Computer
Consultants
1515 Waxhaw Indian Trail
Waxhaw, NC 28173
(704) 843-2414

Appendix B

Considerations in Selecting a Personal Computer

1. Decide what you will do with the computer.
    Do you expect to use it several hours each day or only on
    occasion? What will you use it for? The answers to these
    questions will help you decide what kind of programs, or
    software, you'll need.
2. Set a budget.
    Figure out what you can afford to spend for everything:
    computer, peripheral hardware, software. Don't forget that
    many advertised computer prices don't include such necessary
    things as a video screen or keyboard.
3. Pick the software.
    Once you know what you want to do, start checking out
    programs that help you do the job. The most important thing is
    to get a good hands-on feel for a program before you buy it.
4. Choose the hardware.
    The selection of software will whittle down the number of
    hardware options for you. You'll need to weigh the speed and
    features of the computer against its cost. The least expensive
    computer, though, may not offer enough room to grow.
5. Visit several computer stores.
    Look for a store that will answer your questions in English, not
    jargon, and that offers service as well as a good price. Some
    brands are available by mail order. You may save money that

way, but you should find out the policies for after-sale support and service because you won't be dealing with someone locally.

Basic Terms to Understand

BIT: The shorthand term for "binary digit," of which there are only two - 1 and 0. It is the smallest piece of information a computer can understand. Some components of a computer are described in terms of the number of bits of information they can handle simultaneously. A 16-bit microprocessor can handle twice as much information at one time as an 8-bit one.

BUS: The electronic "path" by which the CPU exchanges data with add-in circuit cards. The most common bus is the 16-bit ISA, or Industry Standard Architecture design. More advanced 32-bit buses in widespread use are EISA, Micro Channel and NuBus.

BYTE: A unit of information consisting of eight bits. A single byte can represent one letter or number. The amount of random-access memory or the capacity of a disk drive in a computer is expressed in bytes, kilobytes (1,024 bytes), or megabytes (about 1 million bytes) .

CPU: Short for Central Processing Unit. The CPU is the computer's hub that contains most of its basic hardware, including the microprocessor and memory chips. The other parts of the computer, such as the screen and keyboard, are connected to the CPU.

DISPLAY: The computer screen on which you view your programs and data. The least expensive screens are monochrome—usually green or amber characters on a black background.

FLOPPY DISK: Flexible platters coated with a magnetic material used to store programs and data. Programs you buy at the store will also be supplied on floppy disks. They typically hold from 360 kilobytes to about 1.5 megabytes.

HARD DISK: Similar to floppy disks. They are generally permanently installed and hold a great deal more data, usually at least 20 megabytes or more.

MEMORY: Technically, any part of the computer that stores data, including disk drives. Most often, the term refers to the random-access memory chips inside the CPU.

MICROPROCESSOR: The chip that serves as the brain of the computer, whose speed and other attributes generally determine the overall performance of the machine.

MODEM: A device that connects the computer to a telephone line so it can communicate with other computers, including electronic "bulletin boards" and commercial information services.

MOUSE: A palm-sized device that you roll along the desk top to manipulate an arrow on the computer screen. Buttons on the mouse let you control certain computer functions based upon where the pointer is.

RAM: Short for random-access memory. RAM chips in the CPU are used to store the program and data you are using at any particular time. Most modern personal computers have at least 512 kilobytes of RAM; many have 1 megabyte or more.

ROM: Short for read-only memory. ROM chips, programmed at the factory, contain instructions the computer needs all the time. You can't change them.

WAIT STATES: The time during which the microprocessor "waits" to get needed information from slower components.

Appendix C
RIS Checklist (Inventory of Basic Features)
Feature
Patient Management (flash cards, logs, etc)
Scheduling (includes conflict checking)
Quality Control (repeat rates & radiation dosage)
Transcription (with word processor/spell checker)
Film Tracking (track outstanding jackets)
Equipment Maintenance (track downtime)
Inventory (track supply usage and purchases)
Personnel Manager (address/phone book)
Standard Procedures (replaces typed book)
Billing (HCFA forms, aged reports, statements, etc)
Mammography
HISLink (optional HIS interface)
FAXLINK (optional-FAX completed results)

2.2 PICTURE ARCHIVING AND COMMUNICATION SYSTEMS

A Picture Archiving and Communication System (PACS) or IMACS (Image Management and Communication System) is a network of electronic devices connected together with a computer to collect and distribute image data. When first introduced, PACS were considered to be the total imaging management answer for radiology departments (the rate at which radiology would become "filmless" was greatly exaggerated). Hospitals have been slow to adopt PACS technology; it's a situation of too much too fast at an exorbitant price tag.

A total PACS electronic network for collecting, transmitting, viewing, and storing digital images is a global solution for medical image management problems. (See Figure 2.1) Most hospitals see PACS technology as a means to solve specific problems. Going full

Figure 2.1   PACS Electronic Network

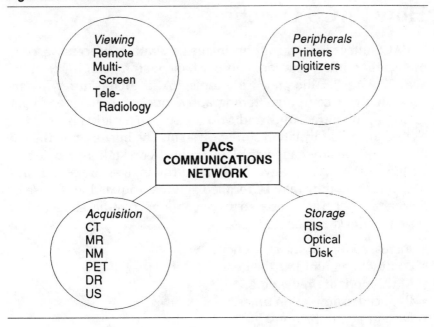

blown filmless is not the immediate goal of most radiology professionals. Manufacturers are responding to the tailored needs of imaging departments by offering application specific technology. For instance, a hospital may determine that image transmission to the emergency room or the ICU is a high priority. Thus, a computer workstation and film digitizer may be employed to link these critical care areas to radiology.

Acceptance of PACS technology has been slow. Radiologists like film, and they are slow to adopt new methods of acquiring and reading images. Because plain film radiography and fluoroscopy accounts for 70 percent of all diagnostic imaging, converting to a digital format in all of radiology would be a formidable and costly endeavor. Vendors recognize the need to overcome these obstacles to PACS acceptance and now emphasize that imaging management and communications can be phased in according to the needs of individual departments. The industry is also hard at work educating radiologists and referring physicians about the potential uses of PACS. The various pieces of PACS that exist today are described in figure 2.2.

How PACS Function

PACS integrate and support image generation, processing, communicating, interpretation, and permanent storage of medical images. Figure 2.3 illustrates a simple PACS architecture. Images generated via computed tomography, nuclear medicine, digital radiography, ultrasound, and MRI are sent in a digital format to a central image information storage system. The images may then be "called up" on any image display console (workstation) that is connected to the PACS network. Because the images are stored in a digital format, they may be recalled and manipulated with ease by the reader. PACS as compared to conventional film-based recording systems offer many advantages:

- Increased diagnostic efficiency.
- Ability to manipulate the image.
- Multi-modality reviewing.
- Reduced examination times.
- Faster patient thru-put.

Figure 2.2   PACS Components

Computed Radiography	Provides for totally digital input from radiography. Consists of a stimulable phospher plate, plate reader and data entry terminal. **Advantages:** Excellent quality images, significantly reduces or eliminates film usage, lessens radiation doses.
In-house Film Distribution Sys.	Allows for images to be distributed within the hospital over a local area network. Consists of a film digitizer, file server and display station(s). **Advantages:** Immediate access to current (and prior) films by the nursing units, reduces film loss.
Optical Archive Sys.	Provides high-volume storage of digital images on optical disks. Media costs comparable to microfilm. Over 100,000 images per disk capacity. **Advantages:** Dramatic reduction in storage requirements. Easy access to prior images.
Radiology Information Sys.	Allows for increased department productivity. Modules include patient scheduling, film tracking, charge capture, results reporting and others. Often interfaced to hospital information system. **Advantages:** Increased charge capture, better resource utilization, reduced turnaround time for reports.
Teleradiology	Allows images to be transmitted over phone lines between hospitals, from hospital to physician's home or from hospital to clinic. Consists of a computer, high speed modem, image capture and display boards, and image processing and transmission software. **Advantages:** Provides for rapid preliminary diagnosis from remote site(s), time savings.

Source: Adapted from *Healthweek*. June 11, 1990.

Figure 2.3   Simple PACS Architecture

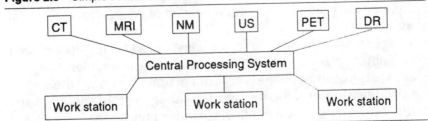

- Online access to previous studies.
- Reduction in lost films.
- Simultaneous viewing.

PACS Components and Subsystems

Data Compression describes the technique used to reduce the amount of information that must be archived and managed by the PACS. Compression is the process of reducing the amount of data it takes to represent an image. The amount of compression could reach a ratio as high as 40:1. Compression ratios in the 2.5:1 range are used without loss of original data and degradation of image quality. The higher the compression ratio, the greater the loss of image integrity. A major problem with compression is that nondestructive compression methods don't really save much disk space. Destructive compression methods result in a loss of high frequency information that adversely affects image quality and diagnostic value. The two main benefits of compression are faster transmission of images and greater storage capacity. Compression remains a serious issue to consider in evaluating PACS technology; the legal ramifications of discarding diagnostic information for space savings is a real concern.

Image Archiving of CT, NM and MRI on tape or floppy disks now approaches the same logistical nightmare of conventional film storage. Current archival methods of these modalities are manual, time consuming, and expensive. The retrieval process is slow and the incidence of filing and refiling increases the rate at which these records are "out of file." PACS' use of optical and magnetic recording devices make storage of digital images cost competitive with film. The PACS acquires images directly from the host computer, and they may be printed on a soft copy medium or dispatched to a laser printer for hard copy film. The intangible benefit is access to previous or complementary studies without the delay of conventional archival methods.

Image transmission or "teleradiology" is the term that describes the capability of sending an image from one site to another. The time it takes to transmit an image is dependent upon the size of the image, the compression of the data, and the mode of transmission. Currently, transmissions are made via standard telephone lines, micro wave, and satellite.

Local distribution networks are one example of putting teleradiology to practical use. Selected images from radiology are sent to physicians in intensive care units and emergency rooms. These local distribution setups are often hard wired together and do not rely on telephone lines. Image transmission technology is also used for the radiologist on call. Sending the images to the radiologist's home is a way to get a preliminary diagnosis and the expert opinion of the radiologist. Over 1,000 teleradiology systems are in place in the United States; most connect on-call radiologists to their host hospital.

Workstations where images are manipulated and displayed commonly have such features as windowing, leveling, magnifying, and 3D reconstruction. Workstations will perform in terms of speed and resolution depending on application. The cost of these display stations will differ according to their performance requirements such as retrieval speed, resolution, and number of display screens.

Pros and Cons of PACS

Pros

- Allows immediate access to images and related information.
- May be used by multiple readers at different locations simultaneously.
- Images in digital form have the potential to improve diagnosis via image enhancement methods.
- Has the ability to display different images from multiple modalities aiding the reader in comparing findings of complementary studies.
- Communication and access to patient information improves with the use of local networks.
- Reduces dependency on film for primary diagnosis.
- Can reduce film costs and associated handling costs (space, filing, etc.).
- Enhances on-call service of radiologist.
- Facilitates the management of teaching files and interesting case studies.
- PACS and RIS integration promotes better department management.
- Reduces exam time for the patient; reduces repeat rates with imaging processing.
- Improves perceptions of service from radiology by the clinician by assuring quick access to clinical information and image review.

Cons

- PACS are expensive; cost savings are difficult to quantify in smaller institutions.
- PACS integration is difficult; PACS/RIS/HIS interactions are problematic.
- ACR-NEMA Digital Imaging and Communications standards are still being phased into current PACS configurations.
- Radiologists like film and the reassurance film offers as a material substance.
- Radiologists are concerned that too much access to medical images by other clinicians will result in a bypassing of the radiology consultation.
- As with all electronic equipment, a controlled environment with attention to temperature, ventilation, and humidity must be maintained.
- PACS transmitted images require more careul evaluation than filmed images according to some radiologists, and usually require manipulation before a confidence level for monitor interpretation of images is achieved.

Conclusion

It seems that the humble beginnings of image transmission via teleradiology systems is spreading the RIS/PACS/IMACS bug to once skeptical users. Although the touch and feel of x-ray film is still near and dear to the hearts of radiologists, now that more than 5,000 teleradiology networks exist, the concept of soft copy interpretation of images from a video screen is almost commonplace. While commonplace is a bit of an over statement, one expert predicts that routine soft copy interpretations are a decade away. What will the PACs environment be like in the year 2000?

RIS/PACS/IMACS will become affordable. That is, PACS technology will be sold in configurations to users that meet the current needs of the buyer. Built-in expandability, flexibility and upgradeability necessary to get bigger and better as time and requirements dictate will be a boiler plate specification.

RIS/PACS/IMACS will get fast. Primarily complaints about PACS systems by radiologists are that they have to wait too long for images.

Fast image display with ease of callback of previous and complementary studies will be a standard feature of every system. RIS/PACS/IMAC will never be as fast or easy as flipping x-rays up one at a time on an x-ray film viewer, however, the expense and the effort of moving heavy x-ray film jackets around will be a welcome tradeoff.

RIS/PACS/IMACS will add FTEs instead of reduce them. By the year 2000 PACS operators will become so specialized that they will have their own complex hierarchy of training, cross training and career ladder tracks that will leave the average manager wondering what these highly technocratic personnel are doing. Take a lesson from the evolution of current information systems. RIS/PACS/IMACS will need applications specialists, key operators, programmers, program analysts, and customer representatives.

RIS/PACS/IMACS will steal the mystery from imaging. With teleradiology networks, online capability to manipulate images and the ability to call up any image at any time and compare it with other modalities makes a trip to the imaging department for a consultation with the radiologist a rare event. It's going to be lonely down there in the place where they used to take x-rays. No more film to handle, just technologists and radiologists fiddling knobs and turning dials at video screens.

The ACR-NEMA Digital Communications Standard will finally be a reality. At last, there will be compatibility among the dozens of imaging systems on the market.

Hints for Hastening the Future

According to Rob Hard of *Hospitals* magazine, hospital executives contemplating the selection of information systems need to link the vision for an information system to the hospital's overall strategic plan. Systems selection should be based on the benefits that will be accrued by the hospital. Key decision makers need to be aware of the hospital's overall strategic plan for information management so that a radiology system makes good operations sense for the organization. A process whereby objective decision-making can occur needs to be set in place to insure that a system selection has not been influenced by any conflicts of interest that do not coincide with the hospital's plan. Hard also writes that a system that involves patient data, results reporting and medical records needs to have medical staff involved in the selection process. The needs of the medical staff need to be reviewed carefully before a decision is made about RIS/ PACS/IMACS.

Howard Schwartz, FAHRA, of the University of Minnesota Hospital presented a perspective on the current RIS environment at a 1992 RSNA refresher course. From a clinical practice and business sense, he suggests that RIS/PACS/IMACS decisions be based on some basic objectives.

1. Look at the reasons for automating manual functions and image transmission in radiology.
2. Consider the state of the art in radiology information systems and PACS concepts and decide whether or not the technology yet exists in order to meet the needs of your organization.
3. Understand that systems may be configured in both integrated and interfaced architectures.
4. Know the pitfalls associated with the selection and installation of these complex information and image transmission systems.
5. Prepare an implementation strategy for your PACS/RIS/IMACS needs. In particular, explore hospital and physician networking issues.

Dr. William R. Brody of the Johns Hopkins University in Baltimore recently offered a list of questions to ask before purchasing a RIS/ PACS/IMACS. Dr. Brody suggests that a great deal of wisdom was gained through making many mistakes with their PACS system at Johns Hopkins. To help others avoid those mistakes he suggests these questions:

• How will scanners be interfaced to the system? Analog interfaces may contribute to degradation of the image.
• How will images be transferred from the various parts of the RIS/ PACS/IMACS system? How long will it take to transfer the images from one place to another?
• How will the images be stored? Can stored images be moved from one workstation to another?
• Will resolution on screens at PACS workstations be good enough? Will the workstations be fast enough?
• How user friendly will your RIS/PACS/IMACs system be? Will the equipment be compatible with future versions of the computer hardware and software from the same vendor?

- How secure will your data be? Is there a safeguard against loss of information due to power failures, crashing disks or lightning bolts?
- How many people will it take to run the system? How much maintenance will be required and how will hardware and software upgrades be handled?
- Can the system easily be made bigger? How many users will the system accommodate at one time and how much image storage will be kept on line? Finally, will the RIS/PACS/IMACS system and RIS system interface?

Appendix A—PACS in Place in the United States*

Supplier	Location
AT&T/Phillips	North Carolina Baptist/ Bowman Gray School of Medicine, Winston-Salem, North Carolina
	Duke University Durham, NC
Advanced Video Products	Veterans Administration Hospital, Iowa City
	Downstate Medical Center/ Kings County Hospital, Brooklyn
DuPont	University of Virginia, Charlottesville, VA
	Shands Hospital, Gainesville, FL
General Electric	Milwaukee County Medical Complex, Milwaukee, WI
Genesys	Jackson Memorial Hospital, Miami

*Adapted from *Diagnostic Imaging: Focus on PACS*. September, 1990.

Siemens	Regional Medical Center, Memphis
	Vanderbilt University, Nashville
Vortech Data	Magnetic Resonance Institute, Boca Raton, FL
	Johns Hopkins Medical Institute, Baltimore

Appendix B—Glossary of PACS Terminology*

Archiving: Long-term storage of information such as images, documents, and/or digital data in an orderly fashion.

Coaxial Cable: A cable consisting of a central conductor and a concentric shield used for the transmission of voice video and/or data signals; the basic transmission medium for cable television.

Computed Tomography (CT): An image acquisition device utilizing x-rays to generate cross sectional images.

Digital: A numerical representation of discrete values typically used by computers.

Digital Radiography: An image acquisition process which yields radiographic images in digital form.

Digitizer: A device which converts a continuous signal or value into digital form (e.g., film digitizer).

Hospital Information System (HIS): A computer system designed to support the operations of the complete hospital. Typical functions include billing, registration, order entry, pharmacy information, laboratory information, medical records, etc.

Image Acquisition Device: A device used to obtain an image which is introduced into a PACS (e.g. CT, MR, Digitizer).

---

*Adapted from *PACS: A NEMA Primer*. 1988.

Image Processing: Any operation performed to enhance or clarify an image for easier diagnosis.

Information Management System: A computer system within a PACS designed to keep track of all image and related patient data.

Jukebox: A device which contains a number of disks or tapes for archival purposes and has the capability to retrieve a specific disk when requested.

Leveling: Refers to adjusting the average intensity (brightness) of the image displayed on the screen of a workstation.

Magnetic Resonance (MR): A modality which applies a high magnetic field and creates images by using the differences in magnetic properties of the atoms in a patient.

Modality: A diagnostic technique, usually intended to create an image either digitally or on film. Digital modalities are, for example, CT, MR, Nuclear Medicine, and Ultrasound.

National Electrical Manufacturers Association (NEMA): An organization supported by its members and active in standardization and regulatory affairs.

Optical Disk: A medium that uses laser energy to store and retrieve digital data (comparable to a compact disk in consumer electronics).

Radiology Information System (RIS): A computer system designed to support the operations of the radiology department. Typical functions include exam order processing, exam scheduling, patient tracking, transcription, reporting, film tracking, and billing.

Viewing Station: An electronic device for the display of text and medical images in digital format; generally used for review.

Windowing: Refers to adjusting the range of intensity (brightness) displayed on the screen of a workstation.

Workstation: An electronic device for the display, manipulation, and evaluation of text and medical images in digital format; usually for diagnostic purposes. It consists of one or more display monitors and some means of user interaction with the system (i.e. keyboard or mouse).

2.3 WRITING EQUIPMENT SPECIFICATIONS

It is estimated that more than 130 million people receive diagnostic radiologic examinations each year in the United States. Manufactured radiation-producing devices are responsible for 90 percent of the population's exposure to radiation. In 1968, federal legislation entitled the Radiation Control for Health and Safety Act (PC 90-602) was enacted to reduce patient exposure during radiographic examinations. The previously unbridled use and manufacture of radiation-producing apparatus became a tightly legislated and closely monitored industry. The radiology equipment standard calls for machines capable of serving the public with increased diagnostic accuracy and a greater level of radiation protection.

The standard, which is an equipment performance standard, is aimed mainly at the equipment manufacturer. The standard mandates levels of performance, and it is the manufacturer's responsibility to comply with these standards. The standard applies to systems and components manufactured after August 1, 1974. Major components regulated by the standard must be certified for compliance by the manufacturer and include items such as x-ray tubes, generators, controls, spot film devices, film changers, collimators, image intensifiers, tables and cassette holders.

Acquisition of Equipment

The selection of radiologic equipment is made jointly by the radiology manager, hospital administrator, and the medical director. Each member of this selection team may approach the purchase of the equipment from a different point of view. The radiologist will view the purchase in terms of which equipment best meets the needs of the patients. The radiologist seeks the most accurate diagnostic information that can be acquired. The hospital administrator speaks for what is best for the whole hospital. Control of the institution's purse strings also rests with this individual. Assuring the efficiency of the department is the responsibility of the radiology manager. Generally, the equipment specifications are reviewed by the radiology manager and radiologist, and the financial details are arranged with the hospital administrator or comptroller.

Radiology equipment is so expensive that acquiring it is a serious undertaking. It is procured by two methods: purchasing or leasing. Directly purchasing equipment is the least expensive alternative. Unfortunately, small hospitals do not have the resources to commit to radiology equipment, but they need this expensive equipment to provide quality patient services, maintain competitiveness, and retain professionals.

The Economic Recovery Act of 1981 provided changes in the tax laws that encourage institutions to use leasing arrangements to acquire expensive equipment. Leasing equipment has some attractive features for hospitals. Technology is changing so rapidly that obsolescence is a major concern. Leasing allows the flexibility of upgrading the equipment by adjusting the terms and payments of the lease. With leasing, a large outlay of cash is not made and the cash flow of the institution is not affected. Leasing also allows for third-party reimbursement on the costs of renting the equipment. The rental costs are considered part of the hospital overhead. It is important to understand that a lease for the purpose of third-party reimbursement provides for renewal or purchase of the equipment for fair market value at the end of the agreement.

Prepurchase Considerations

The radiology manager must consider the design and utilization of physical facilities before purchasing major equipment. It is obviously a mistake to commit the hospital to a purchase without the vendor providing schematics illustrating the appropriateness of the equipment for the space provided. Careful review of the proposed layout plans will eliminate future problems, such as collisions between equipment suspended from the ceiling and fixtures in the room. A maximum ceiling height should be determined to avoid focal film distance limitations and electrical requirements must be adequate to support the equipment. The electrical supply for modern x-ray equipment is usually 208 to 230, or 480 volts. Most radiology departments have electrical service provided by a dedicated transformer. If a new transformer is needed, 480-volt service is preferred because it is less expensive than 208-volt service. A final prepurchase consideration is the total weight of the system. The weight-bearing capacity of the building for the proposed equipment should be evaluated by a structural engineer.

Equipment Specifications and Performance Standards

In a general sense, the radiology manger knows what the equipment requirements are for the radiology department. However, considering that the purchase of equipment is a choice that will have to be lived with for several years, a little homework concerning the kind of equipment being sought is in order. First, it must be decided what is needed. Some elements to consider when determining equipment requirements are the patient, the clinician, and the setting for the proposed service. The radiology manager, the radiologist, and the hospital administrator can draw from experience and acquaintances with other professionals to make the best selection for the department. This selection will be made after long conversations with equipment sales representatives and close scrutiny of many technical sales brochures. Once available merchandise is surveyed and equipment purpose is determined, technical specifications should be considered, which alone will determine later performance. Technical specifications constitute a language spoken by each of the equipment vendors. Differences will become apparent as comparisons are made of the different equipment proposals based on the same criteria of selections. The bid specification is a chance for the purchaser to specify what is wanted from the vendor. Performance specifications are written into the bid specification as performance criteria.

Preparing Performance Specifications

Performance specifications for radiologic equipment will reflect the users' specific requirements, industry standards, government regulations, and technical specifications to be met by the manufacturer. Performance levels referenced in a specification document should be reasonable; that is, achievable by most equipment manufacturers. Equipment specifications and performance levels that are too specific or restrictive will raise an issue of fairness with the vendors. Too restrictive a set of specifications also limits the number of potential bidders and often drives up the costs of systems by encouraging an environment of overspecifying components that will end up in more costly system configurations. Exceptions to performance specifications, when offered by vendors, are common and should be identified as substitutes and justified as a comparable alternative to the required specification.

A standardized approach to equipment purchase utilizing a performance specifications format is one way to assure that equipment will operate satisfactorily when it is installed in your department. The performance specification method will allow easy comparison of equipment capabilities and thus facilitate a selection of the best system for the particular circumstances that exist at your facility. Once the vendor has supplied the information describing the technical performance of the equipment, you can demand that the equipment performs to those parameters following installation. The final contractual arrangement with the vendor should specify a period and procedure for acceptance testing of the new equipment against its published performance specifications. See appendices to this chapter for examples of equipment performance specifications.

Other Prepurchase Considerations

It is through experience and suffering the pitfalls of leaving just one page unturned that every new equipment purchase is better negotiated, selected, and installed than the most previous one. If you were to assemble a group of radiology managers together to share equipment selection disasters, a long list of perhaps obvious check points would unfold. The following list of purchasing hints may prove helpful to future equipment acquisitions for your facility:

1. Use a physicist or other consultant to construct performance specifications.
2. Include acceptance testing into your bid document.
3. Use an attorney to review all purchase agreements.
4. Get assurance that service on the equipment will be immediately available.
5. Negotiate service training for in-house engineers at no cost.

6. Negotiate service contracts at point of purchase at substantial discount.
7. Arrange for extended warranties.
8. Specify total installation time.
9. Insert penalties for late delivery, extended installations or periods of initial nonperformance according to equipment specifications.
10. Specify maximum response time for service requests.
11. Insist on free telephone consultation for repairs.
12. Limit travel time paid to vendor service personnel to one hour.
13. Require that vendor supply any necessary spike suppression for incoming electrical power.
14. Request free software upgrades and discounts on add-on technology.
15. Arrange for free operator training at the factory (if necessary) to include tuition, travel, and lodging.
16. Specify on-site vendor supplied operator training for technologists and physicians.
17. Negotiate guarantees on maximum tube life and free replacements.
18. Arrange to bill the cost of repairs back to the vendor for extended periods of downtime.
19. Specify that costs of shipping and installation be the responsibility of the vendor.
20. Request input into the selection of the local service representative assigned to your facility.
21. Request that the vendor assist with interim service (e.g., CT, MRI during the installation period).
22. Require that a complete set of schematics and operator's manual be provided at no charge.
23. Negotiate more favorable terms for the hospital, a smaller down payment, and a greater final payment conditional upon final acceptance.
24. Specify that the warranty period begins at final acceptance, not installation date.
25. Specify that the vendor is responsible for delivery of the equipment from your loading dock to the installation site.
26. Require that the vendor dispose of all waste and packing materials.

27. Negotiate with the vendor to shorten installation time by working weekends and extended hours at no charge.
28. Preplanning for the installation should include:
    a. Access to installation site. Check size of corridors, elevators and weight restrictions.
    b. Power requirements. Is power available for the new equipment?
    c. Water service, to include any special pressure requirements
    d. Medical gases, and
    e. Adequacy of air conditioning to support new equipment (often a problem in older buildings).

Appendix A

Sample Equipment Specifications for a Radiographic/Fluoroscopic Room. Illustration Courtesy of Pete Bartolazzi, Appleton, WI.

SAMPLE EQUIPMENT SPECS FOR FLUOROSCOPIC ROOM

Generator:
1. 3 Ø or high frequency generator
2. 600 MA
3. 150 KVP
4. 50 to 150 KVP in stops of 1 KVP
5. MA 50 to 600 (state MA stations)
6. Solid state timer, m/s to 6 seconds
7. Solid state contracting
8. Constant load or constant potential
9. State power requirements
10. 60 KW rating
11. State maximum MA at 1/10 sec. at 100 KVP
12. High speed rotor, 10,000 rpm
13. Microprocessor programmable

Performance specs of above generator: same
Table:
1. 90–30 tilting table
2. 4–way power flat top table—state longitudinal and transverse travel

3. Foot board
4. Patient restraint strap
5. High speed Bucky
6. 12–1 Bucky grid, 103 line ultralum, 48" to 40" focus
7. Table top center stop
8. Table angulation horizontal stop
9. 3–field automatic exposure control
10. Table top to Bucky tray distance

Spot Film Device:
1. 11 X 14—10 X 12—9 1/2 X 9 1/2 cassette sizes
2. Front load—auto
3. 12–1 spot film grid, 103 line ultralum
4. Multiple film format:
   1 on 1   3 on 1   11 X 14
   2 on 1   9 on 1   mini spot
   4 on 1
5. Spot film location indicator
6. Automatic location of mixing film formats
7. Automatic coning to spot size selected
   (preferable servo drive shutters)
8. State time delay from spot film initiation to exposure
9. Triple detector automatic exposure control
10. Fluoroscopic protection apron

Radiographic and Fluoro Tube:
1. 3.5" anode, 350,000 heat unit storage
2. 10,000 rpm
3. .6 mm, 32 KW, 1.2 mm, 60 kW focal spots,
   12–degree angle for field coverage

Tube Hanger:
1. Overhead 3–D ceiling mounted tube hanger
2. Electronic locks
3. State vertical, horizontal and transverse travel
4. Vertical detent 48"
5. Horizontal detent 114" and 48"
6. Center detent to table and vertical cassette holder

Image System: TV System
1. 4"–6"–9" high–resolution image tube (state gain and resolution
   characteristics)

2. 510 line TV monitor with automatic brightness control with manual override (prefer fixed KVP fluoroscopy)

NOTE: If the written specification is nonapplicable for your equipment, please state your specifications on a note on how you meet the specification needs.

Appendix B

Sample Equipment Specification Parameters Evaluation. Courtesy of Pete Bartolazzi, Appleton, WI.

SAMPLE

List each parameter stated in equipment specifications and performance specifications. Then, from bid sheets, list each manufacturer in the form of a matrix against each specification. When you are finished, you actually should be able to compare "apples and pears."

For example:

	Vendor A	Vendor B	Vendor C
Generator:			
1. KW	80	80	70
2. KVP range	45–150	40–125	50–125
Tube:			
1. Focal spot size	1mm–2mm	.6mm–1mm	.6mm–1.2mm
2. Focal spot KW	30 KW	40 KW	35 KW
Table:			
1. Top length	72"	84"	76"
2. Top width	30"	34"	36"
3. Longitudinal travel	40"	44"	36"
Performance Standard:			
1. KVP accuracy	±5 KVP	±3 KVP	±3 KVP
2. Low contrast performance	3% at 80 KVP	2% at 80 KVP	2% at 80 KVP
Number of BRH variances	1	0	2

The sample given is not necessarily factual but just a demonstration. But when you are finished, you should actually be able to compare "apples and pears."

Appendix C

Sample Addendum to CT Purchase Order. Courtesy of Pete Bartolazzi, Appleton, WI.

SAMPLE ADDENDUM TO CT PURCHASE ORDER

1. Delivery *(date)*
2. Service training for one *(hospital position—bio–med tech, for example)*, tuition-free, must be completed before the end of one-year warranty or warranty will continue until training is completed.
3. Four weeks installation time.
4. *(Vendor)* will help schedule CT mobile unit for *(hospital)* for entire duration of installation.
5. *(Vendor)* will guarantee no more than $110,000 per year cost of CT tubes, averaged every two years.
6. *(Vendor)* will prorate the generator for five years.
7. Five-day on-site original application training and one two-day follow-up one month after original training.
8. CT scanner will not be down longer than 12 hours due to parts availability or the service will be done at no charge to *(hospital)*.
9. Equipment must pass safety and performance inspection and comply to manufacturer's specifications prior to acceptance. Two operators and one service manual complete with schematica, parts lists, PC board layouts, circuit description, operation theory, troubleshooting, maintenance and calibration data must be furnished. Equipment must have approved hospital-grade electrical power connections. Warranty commences when equipment is accepted for service. Payment authorization will be made when conditions are met.
10. Terms: $50,000 down payment with order, 80% upon delivery, balance upon completion of installation and mutual acceptance testing by *(vendor)* and *(hospital's)* physicist. All operating specifications quoted by *(vendor)* must be met.
11. *(Vendor)* must have a valley-based *(name of equipment)*-trained serviceman. Must respond to on-site service within four hours. *(Hospital)* will pay only one hour total travel per service request. There will be no charge for telephone consults.
12. *(Vendor)* will service the CT computers and bill only by *(vendor)*.

13. This order is contingent on approval of *(the board of directors or appropriate officials).*

Signature of
hospital representative

Signature of
vendor representative

Appendix D

*Keeping Your Peaches from Turning into Lemons**

Caught in the midst of an emotionally charged imaging equipment purchase? Those in charge would be well-served to follow the advice of the late 19th Century British dramatist Oscar Wilde, who, incidentally, is much in agreement with Philip A. Femano, Ph.D., president of **Medical Imaging Consultants Inc.** of West Paterson, N.J. Wilde said that a cynic is someone who knows the price of everything and the value of nothing. Femano says buyer beware and recommends keeping the following items in mind.

- Like any sensible shopper, it's important for hospitals to scrutinize the price tag and be diligent about comparison shopping for systems.
- However, it's just as important, if not more important, to determine the *cost* of the equipment. A good way to determine cost is to divide price by the "useful life" of the device. Five years is a good rule of thumb.
- Renovation costs associated with new equipment should be accurately assessed and budgeted for. This can fluctuate widely depending on the vendor system selected.
- The need for third-party accessories, such as computer workstations, must be considered. Some big systems come with just one operating console and you may require a second console that may or may not be included in the original package.
- Administrators should look at what other project management or technical and medical consultants are needed to complete a project. When there's no one pulling everything together, installations can take months.

---

*Curran, C. Telling it Like it is: Consultants Speak Out. *Second Source Imaging*. 8(3):52, 1993.

- Get the vendor to lock in its service rates, including overtime, for five years. But be sure there's a 30-day escape clause.
- Guard against purchasing a system that gives more high-tech, high-priced horsepower than needed.
- Be wary of me-too talk instead of cutting-edge research when discussing the vendor's upgrade strategy.
- Don't let the vendor get away with answers like, "That's proprietary information," when you ask questions about how much to budget for upgrades over the next five years. Hospitals have every right to know what they need to spend to keep their equipment state-of-the-art.
- If your vendor's lips are sealed on that one, at least get them to commit to a fair-market, trade-in value for the equipment after five years. If things don't turn out as wonderful as expected, the hospital has some protection against today's high-tech peach of a system turning into tomorrow's lemon.
- Call references. Years of grief can be avoided by picking up the telephone and questioning past customers on the uptime, service and image quality of the equipment you're thinking of purchasing. It's particularly helpful to get testimonials from customers who are serviced by the same regional service staff fixing your equipment.

2.4   MOBILE TECHNOLOGY

Since the late 1970s, mobile healthcare has expanded at an astounding rate. It is estimated that there are nearly 1,000 mobile units of all descriptions now in operation throughout the United States. Virtually every community now has access to high technology healthcare via mobile units. These units house diagnostic and therapeutic modalities that are both invasive and noninvasive. Computed tomography has been a real mobile phenomenon, bringing initially very expensive technology to a relatively large outpatient market. As computed tomography (CT) has become more affordable to acquire by providers, the prevalence of CT as a mobile leader is shrinking to a growing MRI market. Other imaging technologies are commonly found on the road. Mammography, ultrasound, nuclear medicine, angiography, lithotripsy, and cardiac catheterization have evolved quickly as mobile services and are increasing accessibility to technology by hospitals and patients. These units enhance an institution's visibility in a community and very importantly keep patients in their hometown for their healthcare.

Why Mobile?

Often a mobile unit is the only means available to a provider for acquiring a new technology. A mobile unit can enable a hospital to implement a new service almost immediately. In the case of lease arrangements, the feasibility of whether the volume exists to support a permanent arrangement can be conducted without that initial costly outlay. If construction costs are prohibitive, if no space is available in existing physical plants or if time is needed to erect a permanent site, then the mobile option is very attractive. Mobile units also offer great flexibility in responding to patient volume. Should expected procedure volumes never meet anticipated levels, mobile units can be used at other sites to maximize utilization. For many small institutions, sharing a unit is the best means of affording a new high technology service.

In states where the Certificate of Need (CON) Process is still in place, frequently mobile technology is excluded from review. This is a very attractive shortcut to establishing a new service for hospitals. Additionally, being able to demonstrate that two or more providers will share a mobile unit shows effort to distribute services in a cost efficient manner. The CON process views very favorably efforts to serve the greatest number of people with the most efficient utilization of healthcare dollars. Shared mobile services easily fit CON mandates to distribute medical services among the population in an efficient and beneficial manner.

Advantages and Disadvantages

Mobile technology has several advantages over the operation of fixed site. They are:

1. Ability to serve multiple locations.
2. Less start up costs.
3. No allocation of permanent space.
4. Access to short-term service.

5. Ability to experience market demand prior to a permanent commitment.
6. Opportunity to work with a turn-key provider.

A careful review of financial considerations and quality of care issues is advisable before implementing a mobile service. Most of the disadvantages of mobile versus fixed-site operations will stem from financial and operational concerns. Some of the disadvantages may be:

1. Higher operating costs per unit of service.
2. Inappropriate referrals.
3. Scheduling problems.
4. Cramped quarters and minimal storage.
5. Technical limitations.
6. Transient personnel.

Where CT, MRI, ultrasound, and mammography are ideal "for the road," the requirement for inpatient ancillary support will limit the practicality of initiating mobile cardiac catheterization or lithotripsy in many instances. It is important to address the clinical appropriateness of some modes of mobile technology and to determine whether a temporary stationary unit adjacent to the hospital is in the best interests of patient care.

Financial Concerns

There are two major financial aspects to consider when conducting the feasibility to launch a mobile technology service. The acquisition costs for mobile units are as varied as the types of mobile services available. The purchase or lease decision will depend on the economic condition of the host hospital, and the option to deal with a mobile service company offers additional financial flexibility. Determining revenues for the service is dependent upon reimbursement. The third-party reimbursement position on the technology you propose to offer should be carefully researched.

Acquisition Costs

The one major difference in acquisition costs for mobile service from that of a fixed installation is the mobile environment. Estimates on the costs of these specially outfitted vans and trailers will vary according to the technology to be housed in them. For computed tomography, the mobile environment could be purchased for near $295,000; a cardiac catheterization laboratory will be close to $425,000. The differences in these environments have to do with the complexity of the equipment, the personnel needed, and the patient support items desired for safety and quality of care. The following items are cost considerations that will need close attention during the planning process for a proposed mobile service:

1. Site preparation.
2. Electrical power requirements.
3. Water and sewage.
4. Waiting and changing areas.
5. Recovery room.
6. Preparation and storage.
7. Access (a jetway to ensure safe transit).
8. Power surge protection.
9. A driver.
10. Purchase versus leasing.
11. Contract management.
12. Signage.
13. Marketing/promotion.
14. Fuel costs.
15. Staff transportation.
16. Film processing.
17. Emergency procedures.
18. Telephone.

Planning ahead (i.e., allowing at least eight to twelve months lead time) will assure the time to consider the many steps and elements that contribute to start-up expenses. You will need to conduct market research, funding, equipment selection and purchase, in-house and outside professional coordination, staffing, accreditation (when indicated), and promotion.

Reimbursement Issues

The first thing a manager should check is the reimbursement status of the procedures to be performed in the mobile setting. Reimbursement is generally not dependent upon whether the procedure is performed in a fixed or mobile setting. Mobile units are prime targets for new technology, and as the manager you will need to ensure that the technology is approved by the Food and Drug Administration (FDA). Without FDA approval, most third-party payers will not reimburse a facility for procedures classified as investigational. Crucial, too, will be a review of your charge master (price list with CPT codes) with a reimbursement specialist. There will be specific policies and regulations operating in your geographic area that will affect third-party reimbursement procedures. Your financial advisors should be aware of these reimbursement variations, as well as understand how third-party payers view ownership of the unit (hospital, physician group, or other organization).

Where to call with reimbursement questions

PET. The Institute for Clinical PET answers queries about PET reimbursement and supplies a computerized database list of insurers that have paid for scans. Contact J. Michael McGehee, executive director, ICP, 2105 National Press Building, Washington, DC 20045; 202/466-4274.

MRI/MRA. The American College of Radiology supplies information on correct coding for reimbursement of imaging procedures, including MRA. Questions can be directed to staff in the ACR's Research Division, 1891 Preston White Dr., Reston, VA 22091; 703/648-8900.

Contrast. Squibb Diagnostics staffs a reimbursement hotline for questions about lowosomolar contrast media. A 50-state database includes coverage policy information and diagnostic codes; 800/842-4296.

Five Mobile Technologies

Magnetic Resonance Imaging

All three types of MRI magnets—permanent, resistive and superconductive—can be used in a mobile environment. When planning for a mobile MRI installation, take into consideration the weight of the unit, the strength of the fringe field, the proximity to ferous materials, the cryogen requirements, the water service, the electrical needs, and the ramp up time.

Computed Tomography

The most prevalent mode of mobile technology is the CT scanner. As the price and size of scanners have decreased, interest in mobile units is turning towards interim service arrangements. Short-term installation to ease the strain on providers who are replacing or upgrading their own scanners is common. The affordability of CT today has brought it into the reach of small hospitals, clinics, and doctor's offices.

Mammography

Breast cancer survival rates are directly tied to early detection and this fact has encouraged efforts to conduct early screening with mammography. Mobile mammography programs can be profitable because of low overhead. Also, a mobile program tends to increase utilization by promoting access; it may be positioned in shopping centers and industrial parks, and it allows women to be examined conveniently.

Lithotripsy

The first mobile lithotripsy unit was FDA approved in June 1986. It is estimated that of the half million persons treated with lithotripsy, about 10 percent of the procedures were conducted in a mobile environment. The lithotripsy procedure requires some traditional inpatient style support. First, the unit will need to be close to a cystoscopy room, and anesthesia support is necessary. There must be a clean surgical environment with proper circulation and gases. Lastly, a recovery area is needed to monitor the patients after the procedure.

Cardiac Catheterization

The major concerns surrounding a mobile cardiac catheterization program are access to emergency hospitalization and surgery and quality control of the images. Because patients are already in a serious state of cardiac care, careful screening for the best candidates in a mobile outpatient style setting is common practice. The costs associated with starting a mobile cardiac catheterization are significant due to the special intensive care requirements of the environment and the price of the x-ray equipment.

2.5   POSITRON EMISSION TOMOGRAPHY

PET Technology

Positron Emission Tomography (PET) has been around since the late 1950s and in clinical use on a research basis beginning in the late 1960s. MRI, in contrast, has developed from the early 1980s at an accelerated rate. The development of PET has been slowed by HCFA's failure to authorize payment for the procedure despite PET's well-defined clinical efficacy and safety.

PET will uniquely and accurately study regional function and biochemistry in the body. PET detects the chemical changes that in most diseases precede anatomical changes. PET as an imaging technique detects tiny particles given off by special radioisotopes

---

PET "Snap Shot"[1]

PET's most constant criticism has been its price. The $1.5 million to $3 million scanner needs no special siting requirements but does use radiopharmaceuticals, called label tracers, which are made in a cyclotron. The cyclotron, about 15 feet in diameter and 7 feet high, costs about $2.5 million and needs a specially shielded room with 3-foot-thick cement walls. When you add to that the cost of support staff including a physicist and chemist to create the pharmaceuticals, the annual cost of running a PET center reaches about $1.6 million. Cyclotron sharing and creative financing are helping hospitals that want PET to maneuver around the price barriers until technology lowers the cost.

Expensive radioisotopes similar to the body's chemicals (oxygen, carbon, fluorine and nitrogen), are the key to PET scans. These are labeled with positive charges in the cyclotron by high-energy bombardment. Due to the isotopes' instability, they have half-lives (the time required for one-half the atoms of a radioactive substance to disintegrate) between 79 seconds and 110 minutes. The short half-life reduces a patient's radiation exposure to slightly more than an x-ray and reduces the time of the scan.

Once radiopharmaceuticals are injected into or inhaled by a patient, they become embraced by the body's cells. Inside the cells, the isotope emits positrons, which attract electrons. When the two opposites crash, they annihilate each other and emit gamma rays, or photons, that shoot in 180-degree directions through cell walls, and are detected by the PET scanner.

The photons hit thousands of scanner crystals. They are detectors that translate the photon energy into computer signals, to obtain tomographic images, through a back projection and filter process similar to CT systems. The filtering creates a dot image which is then stored in computer memory.*

---

* Tighe, L.C. PET: When Will it Get Here? *Second Source Imaging.* 7(12):40-2, 1992.

injected into the body. When the radioisotope decays, positively charged electrons (positrons) are released. When the positron and electron collide, they annihilate each other creating an identical pair of gamma rays that travel in opposite directions. This phenomenon is recorded and translated into a useful image using a computer.

The positron emitting isotopes being used clinically are produced with a cyclotron and readily incorporated with numerous physiologic compounds. Rubidium-82 is a positron emitting radioisotope that is commercially available without a cyclotron. Rubidium has a 76-second half life and is used primarily for myocardial blood flow studies.

Clinical Applications

The current applications of PET that provide beneficial diagnostic information are primarily evaluation of tumors, diseases of the brain and the heart. The clinical usefulness of PET shows the following potential applications:

- **Cerebral Vascular Disease:** PET can aid in the management of cerebral vascular disease and stroke.
- **Cerebral Tumors:** PET can be utilized to evaluate and monitor post surgical treatment of tumors.
- **Grading Tumors:** PET allows the clinician to determine the cellular viability and growth rate of tumor tissue.
- **Dementia:** The long-term potential for PET to distinguish different types of dementia is very promising.
- **Epilepsy:** PET can be utilized to identify the exact location of epileptic lesions for surgical intervention.
- **Myocardial Disease:** PET can be used to determine the size and extent of an infarction, as well as the extent of tissue damage around the area of the infarct. It can also be utilized to distinguish viable from nonviable tissue providing a guide for the treatment of patients with either bypass grafts, angioplasty, or anticoagulant therapy. (This technique requires a cyclotron.)
- **Bone Disease:** PET is a good indicator for abnormal cellular development in bone tissue. It is a more sensitive indicator than conventional nuclear medicine for the identification of metastatic disease.
- **Organ Transplant Evaluation:** PET may be used to aid in the monitoring of the body's reaction to transplant.

PET as a Current Clinical Tool

Clinical Applications of PET*

Positron Emission Tomography's uniqueness in biochemical imaging has led to numerous clinical applications.

Neurology

PET imaging has been very useful and has shown many applications in a diagnosis in management of a variety of neurological disorders. One of the most useful clinical areas is the evaluation of epilepsy. PET has the unique ability of identifying the sites and temporal lobes of epileptic foci. Dementia is another area of clinical usefulness. Approximately 50 percent of all people with dementia have Alzheimer's disease. PET has a characteristic pattern of decreased metabolism bilaterally in the parietal cortex in patients with Alzheimer's disease. PET imaging has also shown applications in ischemic cerebrovascular disease, endovascular therapy, and the detection, management and follow-up of brain tumor patients.

Oncology

PET has been shown to be very useful in the clinical management of cancer patients. Some of the practical uses of PET are as a diagnostic tool for staging patients, monitoring tumor response, determining biologic features of tumors that will affect management decisions, and tracing biological tracks and drugs that are important to cancer treatment. PET is able to measure the metabolic changes in tumors during the course of therapy and for making quantitative measurements of the concentrations of anticancer drugs or antibodies in tumor and normal tissue.

Cardiology

PET is showing a significant role in cardiac diagnosis and treatment. With cardiac imaging, we can utilize both generator and cyclotron based radiopharmaceuticals. PET demonstrates a high sensitivity and specificity for detecting coronary artery disease. It has shown a good correlation between PET and quantitative arteriography

---

*Bucci, R. Positron Emission Tomography: Executive Update Administrative Radiology. 12(5):53, 1993.

for the assessment of severity of coronary artery disease. PET is also useful in determining the viability of the myocardium in patients who have had a previous myocardial infarction.

In attempting to forecast the future role of PET, it should be noted that based on current knowledge it appears that the unique qualities of PET when fully developed will be maintained for some time. The rate of technological progress has accelerated rapidly during the past several years. Since 1982, MRI, Digital Radiography, Color Flow Mapping Doppler, Shock Wave Lithotripsy, and interventional techniques such as balloon angioplasty have become commonplace. As each new modality appears, it causes adjustment to other areas, often reducing the use of lower yielding tests. However, there are areas of overlap, and clinicians are prone to use more than one modality to backup or complement their diagnosis seeking.

In seeking one modality over another, the clinician generally applies certain priorities:

- Use of the least invasive technique that will yield the greatest amount of information.
- Selection of the modality with the highest sensitivity and specificity of diagnosis.
- Selection of the method that is easiest to perform.
- Selection of the least costly approach.
- Selection of an approach which provides information that is synergistic with other diagnostic procedures.

Physiologic Tracers needed to operate the typical clinical PET center

Radiopharmaceutical	Application
$^{18}F_2$-deoxyglucose	Glucose metabolism
$^{13}NH_3$ (ammonia)	Cerebral blood flow Myocardial blood flow
$^{15}O_2, C^{15}O_2, H_2^{15}O$	Cerebral blood flow Cerebral blood volume Oxygen metabolism
^{11}C-labeled amino acids	Amino acid uptake in brain
^{11}C-palmitate	Myocardial metabolism
^{11}C-butanol	Myocardial blood flow and perfusion
^{68}Ga compounds	Multiple applicatons (lung, liver, kidney, blood-brain barrier)
^{82}Rb chloride	Myocardial perfusion

PET Is a Costly Technology

PET, in its steadily improving form, will compete very well with other modalities in the neurological and cardiology areas in particular. There is much research and experience with PET, as it has been in existence since the late 1950s. Nevertheless, before reimbursement is commonplace, PET must develop a clinical track record so that it can be justified in specific situations over competing modalities. This requires enough statistical evidence to assure PET's utility in both a cost effective and clinical efficient manner.

PET technology has a huge price tag and may cost as much as $2.5 million each. The positron emitting isotopes injected into the patient during the PET scan have extremely short half lives. Those used clinically are carbon-11, oxygen-15, nitrogen-13, and fluorine-18, which have half lives of 20, 2, 10 and 110 minutes respectively. Thus, an onsite or nearby cyclotron is needed, which is another cost of $1.5 to $2.3 million. With site preparation expenses, a PET operation could have a total price tag of $5-7 million. So, the price per examination is very high. On the average, it is $1,800 for a cardiac study as compared to a SPECT thallium, which yields similar information for $900. In 1990, worldwide installed bases of PET scanners was only 100 machines. See Figure 2.4 for average costs of a clinical PET scan.

Establishing PET charges

According to Mary Wagner of *Modern Healthcare* magazine, recently completed clinical positron emission tomography centers are

Figure 2.4   Average cost of a clinical PET scan
based on procedures at 26 facilities

	Cyclotron	Rubidium	All sites
Hospital-based sites	$1,541	$2,231	$1,679
Freestanding sites	2,404	1,404	2,188
Other sites	1,641	805	1,257
Average cost, all types of facilities	1,749	1,617	1,716

Source: Institute for Clinical PET. 1991

costing $6 million to $7 million. But what are the elements of that cost, and how should charges be structured to cover them? Mathis Frick, M.D., played a key role in developing a clinical PET center at Creighton University Medical Center in Omaha, Neb. Dr. Frick offered the following guidelines on general costs and charges associated with clinical PET, based on Creighton's experience.

- **Setting charges.** One way to do an economic analysis of clinical PET is to calculate the hourly operational costs. Equipment, personnel and supply costs should be divided into fixed and variable components. This is important if a center does research as well as clinical studies, because it will allow the facility to charge different rates for different uses of the equipment.

  Each PET scan takes about an hour to perform. Depending on the number of studies performed per day, a per-hour operating cost can be determined, and that can be used to establish charges.
- **Building and equipment costs.** Currently, a clinical PET set-up costs as much as $7 million. That amount covers the scanner and cyclotron, monitoring equipment for radiation control, computer workstations and other support equipment. Equipment costs are reduced if a cyclotron is shared by several institutions that have their own scanners.
- **Personnel costs.** At the least, a dedicated clinical PET center requires a medical director, an operator for the cyclotron, a scanner operator, a radiochemist/radiopharmacist, a nurse, administrative staff and a maintenance technician. Total personnel costs can range from $200,000 to $600,000 annually. Other costs, such as a building lease, maintenance contracts and utilities, can vary widely, from $150,000 to more than $700,000 per year.
- **Financing costs.** A key consideration in determining costs for establishing a clinical PET center is the cost of money. For example, $3 million borrowed for 10 years costs $420,000 at an interest rate of 7% and $580,000 at 15%. A hospital can reduce capital requirements by getting grant, foundation or donated money; leasing the building or equipment; or, in the case of teaching hospitals, using education bonds.

The experience of Creighton's $5.3 million Center for Metabolic Imaging, which opened in 1989, is an example of one approach to charges. For cardiac studies, regarded as one of the more expensive and time-consuming PET exams, Creighton charges $1,200 for the technical component of the scan, $300 for the radioisotope and $250 for the professional fee per study. If the center performs 250 two scan heart studies and an equal number of brain scans in a year, its total of 750 scans will generate total charges of $1.2 million. Assuming the hospital collects about 50 cents on a dollar's worth of charges, it will receive about $600,000 in its first year, which translates into first-year operating losses of about $500,000.*

At what point in a new technology's evolution does it become a realistic option for a hospital? What justifies a high-priced new device's place among established more cost efficient technologies? Ben Armbruster, product marketing manager for the Nuclear Medicine Division of Siemens Medical Systems states that the "name of the game is referrals." It is important to build a patient base by having the best clinicians and the newest technology. K. Lance Gould, M.D., professor of medicine at the University of Texas Medical School in Houston, operates a PET scanner at the medical center. Dr. Gould believes that hospitals must examine their philosophy of medicine when they are considering new technology. Does the hospital want its physicians to pursue early detection of medical problems or does it want physicians to treat patients after they have become ill? He states that if you want to avoid practicing the "symptom and salvage approach," then new technologies can open whole new avenues of treatment.

Hospitals that use new technology to gain a competitive advantage are taking a costly gamble. Big-ticket technology does not necessarily translate into added revenues for hospitals. If PET scanning is an improvement over existing technology, then eventually HCFA will approve PET for reimbursement. Until that time, reimbursement to the hospital for PET scans must come from cash customers and some private insurers.

---

*Wagner, M. Establishing Pet Charges Requires Identification of Total Costs. *Modern Healthcare*. November 30, 1992. p. 38.

Appendix A

*Keep unique design requirements in mind when planning for PET**

While design requirements vary from project to project, here's a brief planning guide for any institution planning a PET facility, based on the firm's experience.

- **Select the vendor.** The equipment vendor should be selected before the facility is designed because vendors' PET equipment comes in different sizes and shapes. In addition, the vendor selected by the hospital may offer assistance in site planning.
- **Determine space requirements.** PET center planners should compile a list of all spaces needed for efficient operations. The list should include space for the scanner, the cyclotron or generator, patients, staff, and radiochemistry and radiopharmaceutical laboratories. Because PET technology is attracting the interest of medical personnel, additional space should be set aside to accommodate visitors, both near the equipment itself and in meeting and study rooms.
- **Floor plan.** Specifics of layout will be dictated by the special requirements of PET and how the delivery of service is organized. For example, because the active life of some radioisotopes made in cyclotrons is very short—sometimes only minutes—they must be moved quickly from the cyclotron to the radiochemistry lab to the prep room for injection into the patient.
- **Site requirements.** Adequate mechanical, electrical and plumbing service must be available at the site. PET equipment has some specific site requirements that must be factored into any plan. For example, one manufacturer's specifications require the room for the cyclotron to have a minimum clear floor area of 20 by 25 feet. In addition, it specifies that the floor of the room be constructed to bear the weight of the 133,000-pound cyclotron.

---

*Adapted from "Keep unique...for PET" by Mary Wagner from an interview with Philip Klump of Phillips Swagger Associates. *Modern Healthcare*. November 30, 1992.

- **Cost estimate**. After a final design is completed, an accurate cost estimate can be determined. Earlier in the process, however, architects should be able to provide rough estimates of the project's cost.
- **Certificate of need**. Do not seek a certificate of need until after a design plan is completed and a cost estimate is determined. A hurriedly conceived certificate-of-need application can create a tremendous number of headaches for the institution that must live within the constraints it creates.
- **Regulatory agencies**. Depending on the state and city, the project may have to be approved by the health department, Nuclear Regulatory Agency, fire marshal, city zoning department and other state and local agencies. Budget sufficient time and effort.
- **Bidding and construction**. After the construction plan is completed, bids can be sought. Contractors should understand that while a clinical PET facility contains all of the elements of a typical acute-care hospital, it's different from other healthcare projects because of the requirements for delivery and installation of the cyclotron. For example, when a cyclotron is to be lowered through the roof to the installation site, a heavy-duty crane capable of such a load will be needed to do the job.

In addition, the contractor must allow extra time to install the equipment after the building is completed, because PET equipment must be installed in a dust-free environment.

Appendix B—Glossary of PET Terms

Accidental coincidence. The chance overlap of two unrelated events within the coincidence resolving time of the detecting system, giving an apparent coincidence event. The accidental coincidence is a form of background, which will be distributed randomly about the image. These events are usually measured separately and subtracted from the data. Also referred to as **Random coincidences.**

Aerobic glycolysis. Metabolic pathway for glucose to pyruvate, which then enters the tricarboxylic acid cycle. Complete oxidation of a molecule of glucose to 6 molecules of CO_2 and 6 molecules of H_2O yields net production of 38 molecules of ATP. *See Also* **Glycolysis.**

Anaerobic glycolysis. Metabolic pathway for glucose to lactate with net production of 2 molecules of ATP per molecule of glucose. *See also* **Glycolysis.**

Annihilation. An interaction between a particle and its antiparticle in which the particles are converted to electromagnetic energy in the resultant form of photons with a total energy equal to mass/energy conversion given by $E = mc^2$.

Annihilation radiation. The two equal energy 511-keV photons produced when a positron and electron combine and their mass is converted into energy. The annihilation photons are emitted at 180° to one another. A small portion of annihilation occurs when the positron/electron pair (positronium) are not at rest, resulting in a slight deviation from 1800 emission (i.e., range of 0.30 angulation from 1800). The energy, 511.003 keV, is equivalent to the rest mass of an electron.

Bq. Bequerel. The unit of radioactivity in Standard International Units (SI) as one nuclear decay per second. The more common unit for radioactivity is still the Curie (1 curie = 3.700×10^{10} Bq).

BBB. Blood brian barrier. Typically described as the tight endothelial junctions at the capillary wall that restrict transport and diffusion from blood to brain or brain to blood.

Beta particle. An electron emitted from an unstable nucleus of an atom with an excess of neutrons. Strictly speaking a positron (positive electron) is also a beta particle but commonly beta particle refers to the negatively charged electron form of beta emission.

Carrier-added(CA). Typically applies to the amount of nonradioactive compound added to the synthesis of a radiolabeled compound.

Carrier-free (CF). Radionuclide or stable nuclide when not contaminated with any other radio or stable nuclide of the same element.

CBF. Cerebral blood flow. Strict definition is blood flow in units of ml/min. By convention CBF refers to ml/min/g tissue which is more correctly called perfusion (i.e., blood flow per mass of tissue). LCBF refers to local value.

CBV. Cerebral blood volume. Conventionally given in units of ml/g tissue. LCBV refers to local value.

CMRG1c. Cerebral metabolic rate of glucose. LCMRG1c refers to local value and units are μmoles/min/g (units of mg/min/g are also commonly used).

CMRO$_2$. Cerebral metabolic rate for oxygen. LCMRO$_2$ refers to local value and units are μmoles/min/g (units of ml/min/g are also commonly used).

Coincidence detection. The simultaneous or near simultaneous detection of two events such as the two annihilation photons by two detectors.

Coronary flow. Blood flow through coronary arteries (ml/min); phasic with maximum during ventricular diastole.

Coronary flow reserve. Ratio of maximum coronary flow (after a maximum vasodilation stimulus) to resting coronary flow.

Curie (Ci). A unit of activity equal to 3.700×10^{10} nuclear decays per second or 3.700×10^{10} Becquerel ($1 \text{ Ci} = 10^3 \text{ mCi} = 10^6 \text{ μCi} = 10^9 \text{ nanoCi}$).

Dead time. Time during which information is being processed and a system cannot respond to new information.

Electrophile. A chemical species which is an electron-pair acceptor.

Extraction fraction (single pass). Fraction of substrate or tracer extracted from blood to tissue during the first passage through the organ.

FWHM or FWTM. Full width at half maximum (FWHM) or full width at tenth maximum (FWTM) of the line spread function (LSF) or point spread function (PSF) and is usually used to specify spatial resolution of PET systems.

Glycolysis. The metabolic pathway from glucose to pyruvate with a net production of 2 molecules of ATP per molecule of glucose. Pyruvate can then be converted to lactate (anaerobic glycolysis) or enter the tricarboxylic acid cycle (TCA cycle). Complete oxidation of glucose through glycolysis and the TCA cycle yields a net production of 38 molecules of ATP, 6 molecules of CO_2 and 6 molecules of H_2O per molecule of glucose. The pathway of glycolysis and oxidation in the TCA cycle is referred to as **Aerobic glycolysis.**

Half-life (radioactive). For a single radioactive decay process, the time required for the activity to decrease to half its original value.

Ligand. In regard to neuro and cardiac receptor site, any compound or drug (either agonist or antagonist) that binds to the receptor.

LSF. Line spread function. The full spatial response of an imaging system to a line source of activity. The contribution of the imaging device to the resolution of an image is specified by the shape and width of the LSF. *See* **FWHM** and **FWTM.**

Maximum likelihood. A technique for parameter estimation that chooses those parameter values that cause the observed data to be the most likely outcome.

Mean transit time. The average time for tracer molecules to pass through a flow system. It is equal to the first moment of the transit time distribution curve.

MBF. Myocardial blood flow. RMBF and LMBF refer to regional and local values, respectively. Strict definition is blood flow in units of ml/min but conventually defined as blood flow per gram of tissue (i.e., perfusion) in units of ml/min/g.

MMRG1c. Myocardial metabolic rate of glucose. LMMRG1c refers to the local value and units are μmoles/min/g (units of mg/min/g are also commonly used).

Molar (M). Unit of concentration of 1 mole/liter. 1 Molar = 10^3 miliM = 10^6 microM = 10^9 nanoM = 10^{12} picoM.

Mole (m). Defined as Avogadro's number (N) of atoms or molecules (6.023×10^{23} atoms or molecules/mole). Mole = 10^3 milimoles = 10^6 micromoles = 10^9 nanomoles = 10^{12} picomoles.

MTF. Modulation transfer function. Fourier transform of the LSF and provides a measure of the fraction of signal amplitude that will pass through an imaging system at each spatial frequency.

MVO$_2$. Myocardial oxygen consumption in units of μmoles/min/g (units of ml/min/g are also commonly used). LMVO$_2$ and RMVO$_2$ refer to local and regional values, respectively.

No-carrier-added (NCA). An element or compound to which no carrier of the same element or compound has been intentionally or otherwise added during its preparation.

Nonspecific binding. Binding to tissue (or filters, glassware, etc.) components other than the receptor and is usually measured by incubating the tissue in a high concentration (100 times the K_D concentration) of unlabeled ligand.

Nucleophile. A species with an unshared electron pair.

OEF. Oxygen extraction fraction. LOEF refers to local value.

OER. Oxygen extraction ratio. Defined as the ratio of the net oxygen equivalent of substrate extracted by tissue assuming substrate is completely oxidized to CO_2 and H_2O (*see also* **Oxygen equivalent**) to the net oxygen extraction by tissue.

Partial volume effect. When a structure is smaller, in any dimension, than twice the FWHM of an imaging system, the structure does not fill the sensitive volume of one resolution element of the system and due to this partial volume effect, the measured activity concentration is less than the true object concentration.

Perfusion. Blood flow per mass of tissue in ml/min/g.

Positron. Positively charged electron (anti-electron) that is emitted from the nucleus of an unstable isotope which has an excess number of protons. The positron will combine with an electron and convert the mass of the electron and positron into electromagnetic radiation of two equal energy 511-keV annihilation photons (*see* **Annihilation radiation**).

Purity, radiochemical. The fraction of the stated radionuclide present in the stated chemical form.

Purity, radionuclide. The fraction of the total activity which is present in the form of the stated radionuclide.

Rad. A unit of absorbed radiation dose. 1 rad = 10^{-2} Joule/kg.

Radiochemical yield. For the radionuclides of a specified element, the yield of a radiochemical preparation, expressed as a fraction of the activity originally present.

Random coincidence. See Accidental coincidence.

Receptor. The component within the cell membrane (or in some cases within the cytoplasm) which recognizes and binds an agonist hormone, transmitter, or drug thereby activating an effector of a biological response.

Recovery coefficient. The ratio of the measured isotope concentration of a structure in an image to the true isotope concentration in the structure. The recovery coefficient is a measure of the ability of the system to make a quantitative measurement of specific structures.

RMBF. *See* **MBF.**

Scatter coincidence. A coincident event in which one or both photons originating from the same annihilation event, and, therefore, can be in true coincidence, are scattered (i.e., deflected) before reaching the detectors. The result of a scatter coincidence is the mispositioning of the event in the image.

Specific activity. The amount of radioactivity of a specific radionuclide divided by the mass of the radionuclide or labeled compound into which it has been incorporated (i.e., mCi/g or mCi/mmole).

Specific binding. The difference between total binding to the tissue and binding that occurs in the presence of an excess concentration of unlabeled ligand (i.e., 100 times the KD concentration). Binding of a compound to a specific receptor as opposed to general solubility or nonspecific binding of a compound in tissue.

Standard deviation. The square root of the variance of a random variable. For Gaussian distributions, 68% of the outcomes lie within one standard deviation of the expected value and 95% lie within two standard deviations.

Standard error of the mean. Standard deviation divided by $n^{1/2}$ where n is the number of observations. It is a measure of the estimated mean from n observations.

Steady state. Rate of a transport or reaction sequence is not changing with time.

2.6 LASERS IN MEDICINE

Laser is an acronym for Light Amplification by the Stimulated Emission of Radiation. Created and harnessed by man, it is many times more powerful than the energy of the sun, yet can be focused microscopically to spot sizes as minute as 20 microns. It is the brightest light existing today; and through its unique properties, it has introduced many exciting and remarkable applications in diagnostic medicine and surgery.

The Laser System

The components of a Laser System are: a power source—a laser medium—an optical resonator or laser cavity—a wave guide. The Power source "pumps" energy into the lasing medium to create what eventually becomes a stimulated emission of photons. These photons become the laser light. The lasing medium may be gas, such as argon; carbon dioxide; or crystal or glass mediums such as YAG. The laser light is amplified with the use of an optical resonator and then the laser light is focused with the use of a wave guide, "a series of reflecting mirrors."

Properties of Laser Light

Laser light has three special qualities that distinguish it from conventional light sources.

1. Laser light is all of one frequency or wave length and, therefore, one color. Thus, the laser beam is monochromatic and very pure.
2. The wave fronts of a Laser beam are precisely in step, or phase through time and space. This process is called "coherence" and allows the beam to be sustained over long distances with little diversion.
3. Coherence provides directionality, or collimation, and this provides for the easy control of focusing of the laser beam on tissue surfaces.

Types of Lasers

Of the many types of lasers, the three common ones used for surgery are argon, CO_2, and the Nd:YAG. Lasers operating in the visible light region, such as argon, are seen by the human eye. Those in the infra red range, such as CO_2 and YAG are not visible. Argon lasers may use a regular wall outlet at 110 volts of alternating current or 220 volts of direct current. Argon lasers are not very efficient. They generally require a water cooling system to control heat generation. A fiberoptic wave guide is commonly used for transmitting argon laser light. It can be hand-held or directed to an endoscope or operating microscope.

The CO_2 laser uses power from a regular wall outlet at 110 volts AC. A system of mirrors within an articulating arm allows focusing and directing the beam to a pencil-like hand piece or through an operating microscope. Since the CO_2 laserbeam is invisible, a helium-neon laser is usually combined with the beam to provide a visible red aiming light.

The YAG laser uses 220 volts of direct current and has a water cooling system. The light may be transmitted through a fiberoptic wave guide to a hand piece or endoscope or focused through an operating microscope.

Principle Clinical Uses

The Argon Laser is used by dermatologists and plastic surgeons to photocoagulate vascular lesions such as portwine hemangiomas and other cutaneous lesions. Ophthalmologists utilize the argon for coagulation of proliferative vessels in diabetic retinopathy and for treatment of detached retina. General surgeons and gastroenterologists utilize the Argon laser through an Endoscope.

The CO_2 laser is regarded as the workhorse of lasers. It is well utilized in burn therapy, dermatology, gastroenterology, general surgery, gynecology, neurosurgery, orthopedics, otolaryngology, plastic surgery, and neurology. The mechanism of action of the CO_2 laser is vaporization: the beam hits the target with extreme precision, resulting in concentrated heat intensity that, in turn, causes instantaneous flash boil and vaporization.

The YAG laser is efficient as a coagulating tool. The ability of the YAG to coagulate the extensive blood supplies in tumors and cancers makes it especially useful in oncology. Through flexible fiberoptics, endoscopy is facilitated in gastroenterology, pulmonology, urology, gynecology and general surgery with the YAG laser.

Percutaneous Laser Angioplasty

Percutaneous laser angioplasty for peripheral disease is becoming a mainstream technique. Limited, however, is the use of laser catheters in the coronary arteries, where navigation is difficult and wall perforation from a stray beam or misguided catheter tip can be disastrous. Nevertheless, coronary results in a limited number of patients have been encouraging, and the prospect of conquering lesions impervious to balloon catheters has spawned a variety of ingenious laser devices.

Whereas balloons merely push vascular lesions out of the way, lasers promise to ablate stenotic or occlusive lesions, even calcified ones. Still, the few laser catheters that have won market approval rely mostly on thermal burrowing and only a little on ablation, and against occlusions create only narrow openings that demand follow-up balloon angioplasty.

Beams from all test medical lasers ablate not only plaque but any other tissue as well, so the task is to deliver energy to lesions without making holes in the arterial wall. The risks of perforation—low in the peripherals but ominously high in the coronaries—are being addressed by clinicians working with manufacturers.

Discussion

By far the most widespread use of laser technology has been in surgery by the vascular surgeon. This is largely due to initial marketing direction and technology development that occurred in peripheral vascular laser angioplasty. With coronary applications and more cardiologists expanding into the peripheral vascular market, laser sales to cardiology are increasing. Radiologists are also expanding into patient contact areas through interventional radiology with the technique of laser angioplasty. "Turf" battles are taking place nationwide in hospitals over laser use. Manufacturers are capitalizing on the confusion by marketing lasers to individual departments. This fractioning effect of laser use is counter to the development of strong and efficient programs that share laser resources.

When multiple departments utilize one laser, problems are certain to crop up with scheduling and the potential of a mobility induced failure of the equipment. The solution to avoid conflict among specialties who desire laser use is the creation of an area where all interested parties have access to the equipment.

A laser angioplasty program can pay for itself within a cooperative environment of cardiologists, surgeons, and interventional radiologists sharing systems. Marketing of the service to create community awareness will enhance referrals and help to increase utilization.

2.7 THE BUSINESS OF MAMMOGRAPHY

Breast cancer is responsible for more than 40,000 deaths per year in the United States. Studies have proven that many of those deaths could be prevented through early detection. These grim statistics are rising to an incidence of nearly 150,000 new cases per year despite educational, public health, and clinical efforts to stem the disease. It is a well-publicized fact that about one in ten women will develop breast cancer during their lifetime. It is estimated that the cost of annual screening of 25 percent of women between the ages of 40 and 50 would cost $402 million a year by the year 2,000.

There is some controversy over the value of screening mammography for women under the age of 50. American Cancer Society guidelines recommend a baseline mammogram between 35 and 39, with subsequent screenings every other year until age 50, then yearly thereafter. Screening mammography has been shown to reduce mortality from breast cancer. Although its impact on various age groups is uncertain, there is still debate on how frequently mammograms should be performed, on the best technique, on the ratio of cost to benefit, and on the question of access to all women.

Screening Is More Than Just Mammography

There are three parties to the screening process; namely, the patient who should complete a breast self-examination (BSE) on a regular basis, the radiologist who interprets the results of the radiographic study, and the primary physician who coordinates the data and manages the clinical care of that patient. Patients need to practice periodic BSE after detailed instruction, the radiologist needs to be well trained in mammographic interpretation, and the primary

Recommended Breast Checks for Most Women*

Age	Breast Self-exam	Clinical Exam	Mammogram
20-34	Monthly	Annually	
35-39	Monthly	Annually	
40-49	Monthly	Annually	Every 1-2 years
50 & over	Monthly	Annually	Annually

*All women are at risk for breast cancer. These are screening guidelines for most women without symptoms and no personal or family history of breast cancer. Always follow your doctor's specific recommendations. If you detect a problem at any time, call your doctor immediately.

physician must perform a good physical examination. Collectively, the BSE, mammogram, and physical examination comprise a quality screening process. Other program components that must be in place in order for a screening program to be significantly effective are: affordability, ease of access, and patient compliance of 70 percent on periodic screening follow-up exam. Further, the most effective programs have rigid quality control, skilled interpretation, informed consent, and clear patient education.

Physician Referral or Self Referral

The main reason women do not submit to screening mammography is because their physicians don't send them. A National Cancer Institute survey recently showed that 80 percent of women who never had mammography would have—if it had been suggested by their physician. The physician is the single most important factor in determining whether a woman has a mammogram. In established screening centers with aggressive marketing aimed at women customers, it has been shown that 85 percent of screening visits are still made on physician referral.

Many facilities that perform screening mammography will accept self-referred patients. Those facilities require that a self-referred individual supply the name of a physician who will receive the report. Typically, a center will also maintain a list of physicians who agree to take new patients in order to insure follow-up. A personal physician is essential to complete the screening process. The clinical part of the breast examination is an essential component of any screening program. Centers that do not accept self-referred patients manage to skirt two problem areas. The first is a medical economic issue. Opposition of primary care physicians to self-referred screening is very common. This bypassing of a doctor's visit is a real economic threat to would-be referring physicians. Second, with a physician referral, the radiologist is relieved of the responsibility for clinical examination and follow-up for breast healthcare. Radiologists who are willing to assume those primary care duties take on added responsibilities such as:

1. Recording of an appropriate history and physical examination of the breast.
2. Patient education to include BSE and discussion of mammographic findings in language the patient can understand.
3. Arrangement of follow-up and referral of patients to other physicians.
4. Requesting and correlating other diagnostic procedures such as ultrasound, aspirations, and biopsies.

What Will Make the Program Successful?

There are some fundamentals of planning and customer relations that will spell financial success for your screening venture. It is apparent that in the case of breast screening centers that the primary customer remains the referring physician.

Prior planning before venturing is the first fundamental for success. It is necessary to know and completely understand from the onset exactly what your customer needs will be. Meeting these real and perceived needs is the purpose of all your marketing efforts directed towards your customer (the physician and the patient). These customer needs translate into four major marketing principles:

- Service (promotion).
- Quality (product).
- Cost (price).
- Convenience (placement).

Customer orientation is a major factor for success in a service-related business. Everyone who works at the center must be friendly, helpful, and caring. The typical patient is more sophisticated and educated; they are a new kind of customer who realizes that alternatives exist for healthcare and providers are actively courting their business. The objective of your marketing activities is to influence consumer choice. The factor that will most impact that choice is *service*. Consider this: everyone knows good service, even if they don't know good healthcare!

The *quality* of the screening program is measured in areas that are more physician directed. For example, the reputation of your radiologist and rapport he develops with referring physicians is one aspect of program quality. The reports need to be timely and informative. For the referring physician, they should answer the clinical question and afford direction for future care of the patient. The technical quality of the films is, understandably, essential to expert interpretations.

It is commonly believed that low *cost* is the key to attracting more screening mammography business. Typical charges for screening mammography nationwide are between $50 to $75. A mammography service is a money-maker. Even at a low price it can bring in other revenues from biopsies and surgery. See figures 2.5 and 2.6 for examples of financial analysis.

"Location, location, location" is the real estate credo that applies in a discussion of convenience. You should place your center where the

Figure 2.5   Proforma Income Statement

Mammography Screening Center			
Income	**Year 1**	**Year 2**	**Year 3**
Exams	15/day	20/day	30/day
Revenue	$337,500	$450,000	$675,000
(@ $75 each)			
Expenses			
Capital[1]			
$375,000	$ 75,000	$ 75,000	$ 75,000
Operating			
Lease	$ 20,000	$ 21,000[2]	$ 22,050[2]
Salaries	55,000	57,750	60,638
Supplies	26,000	27,300	28,665
Repair	11,000	11,550	12,128
Marketing	8,000	8,400	8,820
Utilities	24,000	25,200	26,460
Administrative	36,000	37,800	39,690
Other	18,000 (198,000)	18,900 (207,900)	19,845 (218,295)
Total Expenses	$273,000	$282,900	$293,295
Net Revenues	$ 64,500	$167,100	$381,705

[1] 5-year straight line depreciation schedule
[2] Assume 5% increase in expenses per year

Figure 2.6 Proforma Operating Assumptions

Mammography Screening Center

Revenue Assumptions

Charges	$125.00 per exam
Volume (daily)	
1st month	5
2nd month	8
3–6 month	10
7–9 month	15
10–12 month	22
Year 2–5	30

Expense Assumptions

Variable Costs

Supplies per exam	$6.50
Business office	15% of gross billings
Professional fees	25% of collections

Fixed Costs

Lease	$20,000
Utilities	6,000
Insurances	6,000
Marketing	7,500
Salaries	72,000
Benefits	18% of total wages
Inflation Years 2-5	9% per year

patients are and where the referring physicians are located. Convenience to the customer is the purpose of this exercise. Consider all of the following factors when planning marketing tactics for where you will provide your service.

- Parking.
- Physical location.
- Access.
- Hours of operation.
- Ease of scheduling.
- Waiting times.
- Telephone courtesy.
- Assistance with filing insurance claims.
- Discounts.
- Privacy.
- Confidentiality.
- Literature.

Organizations with Mammography Screening Information

American College of Radiology
1891 Preston Drive
Reston, VA 22091
(703) 648-8910
   In addition to general information, provides statements of policy on treatment and recommendations to the radiologist on handling patients who are not referred by a physician.

American Cancer Society
Professional Education Department
1599 Clifton Road NE
Atlanta, GA 30329
(404) 320-3333

Women's Healthcare Consultants
500 Davis St.
Evanston, IL 60201
(708) 869-1200
   Also provides aggregate data on women's preferences in screening.

National Association of Women's Health Professionals
500 Davis St.
Evanston, IL 60201
(708) 869-1200
   Also provides provider survey information on what hospitals charge, how many patients are screened per hour, and whether results are returned to patients or doctors.

National Cancer Institute
Early Detection Education Program
Office of Cancer Communications
9000 Rockville Pike
Bldg. 31, Room 4B43
Bethesda, MD 20892
(301) 496-6792
   Also provides ideas and resources for developing community programs.

For listings of facilities accredited in your area, contact NCI at:
Cancer Information Service
(800) 4-CANCER, or call your local ACS office.

Mammography Accreditation

The ACR Mammography Accreditation Program was established as a voluntary peer review process. Since 1987, the ACR accreditation process has been recognized as the method for determining quality mammography centers. Some third-party payers are linking reimbursement for screening mammography to ACR accreditation. The ACR accreditation program for mammography offers a way for facilities to demonstrate quality, and it has set quality standards for mammography to insure high quality mammograms at the lowest patient dose.

In 1986, the American Cancer Society established a Breast Cancer Awareness Screening Campaign and a joint ACS-ACR Committee on Mammographic Screening was founded. It was quickly realized that an effective breast screening effort would require high quality studies, low dose rates, and accurate interpretations. These concerns resulted in the development of the ACR Mammography Accreditation Program. In 1987, the first three-year accreditations were awarded. By May 1991, 2,380 facilities with 2,925 units had completed and passed the evaluation process. As of Sept. 1992, 9,200 of the estimated 11,000 mammographic units had applied for ACR accreditation. There are ACR accredited mammography facilities in all 50 states, as well as in Puerto Rico and Canada.

Process of Evaluation

The ACR Mammography Accreditation Program is comprised of four phases: application, phantom image quality and dose, technical evaluation of images, and film processing procedures. The application process is the *first phase* and is a thorough survey of the facility seeking accreditation. Information is collected to include:

1. Practice environment.
2. Training and experience of staff.
3. Equipment specifications.

4. Mammographic techniques.
5. Quality assurance.
6. Medical history.
7. Physical examinations.
8. Reporting procedures.
9. Statistics.
10. Film archival.

The *second phase* is an assessment of the mammographic imaging system using a phantom image and calculation of average glandular dose. A strict set of technical procedures is used during this phase with a phantom specifically designed for this purpose.

The technical evaluation of clinical images is the *third phase* of the process. It is a peer review of two sets of clinical mammograms from each unit desiring accreditation. Each set of films are scored on positioning, compression, exposure, resolution, contrast, noise, identification, and artifacts.

Last, the *fourth phase* is a technical critique of processing methods. Day-to-day stability of processing parameters are assessed using 30 days of quality control logs.

Facilities that meet all the standards of accreditation are awarded a three-year certificate.

Responsibilities for Quality Assurance in Mammography

A review of the guidelines for a mammography quality control program will demonstrate that the radiologist, radiology manager, the medical physicist, and radiographer all have important roles in assuring excellent exam quality. The responsibilities of each of these individuals are described in the following figures adapted from the ACR by Arthur Haus of the Eastman Kodak Company.

Figure 2.7 The Radiologist's specific responsibilities are:

1. To ensure that technologists have adequate training and continuing education in mammography.
2. To provide an orientation program for technologists based on a carefully established procedures manual (described in more detail in the ACR publication referenced here).
3. To ensure that an effective quality assurance program exists for all mammography performed at the site. The radiologist should provide motivation, oversight, and direction to all aspects of the quality assurance program.
4. To select a single technologist to be quality control technologist, performing the prescribed quality control tests.
5. To ensure that appropriate test equipment and materials are available to perform the technologist's QC tests.
6. To arrange staffing and scheduling so that adequate time is available to carry out the quality control tests and to record and interpret results.
7. To provide frequent and consistent positive and negative feedback to technologists about clinical film quality and quality assurance procedures.
8. To select a medial physicist who will administer the QC program and perform the physicist's tests.
9. To review the technologist's results at least every 3 months, or more frequently if consistency has not yet been achieved; to review the physicist's results annually, or more frequently when needed.
10. To oversee or designate a qualified individual to oversee the radiation protection program for employees, patients, and other individuals in the surrounding area.
11. To ensure that records concerning employee qualifications, mammography technique and procedures, quality assurance, safety, and protection are properly maintained and updated in the procedures manual.

Source: **Mammography Quality Control** guidelines American College of Radiology Committee on Quality Assurance in Mammography

Figure 2.8 Radiology Manager's Responsibilities

1. To support technologist training in quality control, including travel required to participate in training.
2. To provide the right testing equipment and appropriate quality control tools.
3. To be sure that technologists have adequate time to perform quality control tests and to do the evaluations.
4. To solicit support of industry personnel.
5. To support the radiologist, medical physicist, and technologists so that they can fulfill the responsibilities outlined here, as established by the American College of Radiology Committee on Quality Assurance in Mammography as well as the states which have quality control programs, keeping in mind that good quality control is cost effective.
6. To consider film processing as a complete system and, keeping this in mind, to purchase combinations of film, chemicals, and processors for which the film manufacturer provides information on processing and quality control.

Figure 2.9   Medical Physicist's Responsibilities

The medical physicist's responsibilities relate to radiation safety, image quality and patient dose. Specific tests that should be performed annually include:

1. Mammographic Unit Assembly Evaluation
2. Collimation Assessment
3. Focal Spot Size Measurement
4. kVp Accuracy and Reproducibility
5. Beam Quality Assessment (Half-Value Layer Measurement)
6. Automatic Exposure Control (AEC) System Performance Assessment
7. Uniformity of Screen Speed
8. Breast Entrance Exposure and Average Glandular Dose
9. Image Quality Evaluation
10. Artifact Evaluation

Appropriate tests will need to be repeated by the medical physicist after replacement of the x-ray tube or other major service to the mammography unit.

Source: **Mammography Quality Control** guidelines American College of Radiology Committee on Quality Assurance in Mammography

Figure 2.10   Radiographer's Responsibilities

The technologist's responsibilities center around image quality and, more specifically, patient positioning, compression, image production and film processing. The specific procedures include:

Daily: 1. Darkroom Cleanliness
                  2. Processor Quality Control

Weekly: 1. Screen Cleanliness
                  2. Viewboxes and Viewing Conditions

Monthly: 1. Phantom Images
                  2. Visual Checklist

Quarterly: 1. Repeat Analysis
                  2. Analysis of Fixer Retention in Film

**Semi-
annually:**   1. Darkroom Fog
                  2. Screen-Film Contact
                  3. Compression

Source: **Mammography Quality Control** guidelines American College of Radiology Committee on Quality Assurance in Mammography

Mammography Quality Standards Act of 1992*

President Bush on October 27 signed into law the Mammography Quality Standards Act of 1992, H.R. 6182, giving the federal government authority to regulate mammography services. The new national standard overrides existing federal, state and private regulations.

Originally introduced by Sen. Brock Adams (D-Wash.) as S 1777 in October 1992, the law requires mammography facilities to obtain a certificate of compliance by October 1, 1994 from the secretary of **Health and Human Services** (HHS) in order to operate mammography equipment, interpret mammograms and process mammography film.

To become certified, facilities must meet quality standards in the areas of equipment, personnel and quality assurance, be accredited by a body (either as a non-profit organization or state agency) approved by the HHS secretary and have an annual on-site survey by a medical physicist, according to the law.

The annual inspections will include evaluation of phantom images, beam quality and average glandular dose. Certification is valid for three years and is renewable.

Among the law's provisions are rules requiring facilities to use dedicated mammography units, establish quality assurance and quality control programs to ensure reliability, clarity and accuracy of interpretation of mammograms and standards for mammography of patients with breast implants and appropriate radiation dose.

The law also instructs HHS to establish a National Mammography Quality Assurance Advisory Committee, which would be responsible for advising HHS on "appropriate quality standards and regulations for mammography facilities," among other duties.

Penalties for non-compliance include monetary fines of up to $10,000 a day and possible closure of the facility.

---

* News Briefs: Bush signs mammography bill. *Second Source Imaging*. 8(1):14, 1993.

The U.S. Senate unanimously cleared the bill on October 7, a day after the U.S. House passed the measure. Legislators have set aside $2.5 million in federal funds for fiscal year 1993 and $12 million for 1994 to pay for the national certification of facilities.

Appendix A

American College of Radiology Medicare Mammography Facility Checklist

According to Nicholas Croce, Jr., Assistant Executive Director of the American College of Radiology in Reston, Virginia, the climate for the national certification of facilities is "in a state of flux and subject to change, since the FDA is currently working on standards for mammography facilities." For up-to-date information on accreditation issues, the ACR operates a toll free number (1-800-227-6440).

In March of 1993, the American Healthcare Radiology Administrators republished with the permission of the ACR a useful checklist meant to assist mammography facility operators in complying with the Medicare mammography regulations. That checklist may be available from the AHRA or one of its members. When determining compliance with current law, you should consult governing HCFA regulations (42CFR-494 et. seq.) and the interpretive guidelines for those regulations. Remember that mammography accreditation is an issue of prime public concern and that legislation will be churning out at a rapid rate.

2.8   TECHNOLOGY ASSESSMENT

Today's healthcare environment presents a significant challenge to managers to determine the most efficient way to allocate resources for new medical technology. Medical technology brings significant health benefits and consumes a large share of the nation's healthcare dollars. As a result, those people involved in making the decisions about what new technologies to purchase need to be better informed.

According to the American Hospital Publishing, Inc., and the Linc Group, Inc., a 1990 survey revealed that the top categories of equipment that hospitals plan to acquire are automated laboratory equipment, **radiography** and **fluoroscopy rooms,** patient monitors, **magnetic resonance imaging, CT scanners,** and **ultrasound**. Ultrasound, with many medical applications, is the most popular imaging modality currently being considered for purchase by most hospitals. (See Figure 2.11) Note the strong emphasis on imaging equipment.

Acquiring new capital equipment with an ability to generate a positive margin on operations is of prime interest to hospital CFOs. Financing equipment acquisitions is becoming increasingly more difficult. This stress on hospital cash flow forces a more selective approach to equipment buying.

Hospitals need to develop technology assessment programs that evaluate whether a particular new technology is an appropriate choice for an individual hospital and its patients. With a focus on helping institutions determine which existing and emerging technologies are the right fit, a meaningful technology assessment involves an analysis of how emerging technologies affect physician practice patterns, hospital operations, and quality of patient care. The potential impact of new technologies needs to be examined from the viewpoint of:

- Patient quality of life.
- Staff productivity.
- Reimbursement.
- Documentation.
- Regulatory requirements.
- Ethical considerations.

Figure 2.11 Equipment at Hospitals

TYPE OF EQUIPMENT	Already Have*	Plan To Acquire*
Ultrasound	1	6
Mammography Units	2	10
Automated Lab Equipment	3	1
Nuclear Medicine	4	8
Scanners	5	5
Patient Monitors	6	3
Radiography & Fluoroscopy Rooms	7	2
YAG Lasers	8	9
Argon Lasers	9	14
Cardiac Catheterization Labs	10	7
Carbon Dioxide Lasers	11	13
Radiation Therapy Equipment	12	10
Ambulances, Vans (Ground Trans)	13	11
Magnetic Resonance Imaging (MRI)	14	4
Cardiopulmonary Bypass Systems (heart-lung)	15	15
Single Photon Emission Computer Tomography (SPECT)	16	12
Lithotripters	17	16
Mobile-mounted Imaging	18	18
Mobile-mounted Lithotripsy	19	15
Helicopters/Air Ambul	20	20
Positron Emission Tomography (PET)	21	19
Mobile-mounted Cardiac Catheter	22	17

*In Rank Order

Source: American Hospitals Publishing and the Linc Group, Inc.

Further, new technology assessment should be helping the buyer decide which emerging technologies will best service the future. Additional considerations in the analytical review process should include:

• Establishing the institution as a clinical leader.
• Improving diagnosis and treatment.
• Be futuristic in application.
• Be cost justified.
• Blend in with existing services and physical plant.
• Further the mission of the hospital.

Determining Clinical Value

Objective measures are necessary for verifying the clinical value of existing and emerging technologies. Exploring the clinical value of a particular medical technology may be facilitated by asking some basic questions in order to assess the efficacy and effectiveness of a new modality. From the viewpoint of diagnostic imaging technology, answers to the following basic questions should be sought at the beginning of a new technology assessment.

1. *Does the new technology do it better than the old?* For example, are MRI images that are more pleasing to the eye, but yield no different information than a CT of the same area, enough justification to acquire an MRI machine?
2. *Is the new technology more accurate in reaching a diagnosis as compared to other available imaging methods?* To determine the answer to this question, an acceptable standard of accuracy needs to be agreed upon. One example would be confirmation by pathological specimen. This area of diagnostic accuracy is a difficult aspect of new technology assessment; it means obtaining objective data to support the decision to buy.
3. *Will the new technology replace the old?* Increased accuracy must be proven in order to effectively replace existing diagnostic methods. Often, new technology offerings become complementary to the tried and true routines.
4. *Will the clinical management of the patient be changed?* If a new technology yields more definitive diagnostic information, will it affect therapeutic intervention?
5. *What influence will the new technology have on clinical prognosis?* The well being of the patient must be affected in some way (i.e., length and quality of life).

According to Mark D. Johnson, an analyst with M.D. Buyline, a Dallas-based company that evaluates high-tech equipment, technology shoppers should consider these crucial issues:

- Objectives. What are your department's objectives for the next 12 months? Which ones require capital investment and equipment acquisition? Do any modalities need replacement? What new modalities or technologies should be added? What exhibits will best address your questions about products or services?

- *Competitive posture.* The success of many health-care institutions depends heavily on the community's perception of them as leaders in technology. High-profile imaging procedures and systems can help build a reputation and are, in fact, used as marketing tools by hospitals. Should your facility expand its service offerings with new imaging modalities and if so, which ones?
- *Return on investment.* Adding a new procedure or device to an imaging department requires capital expenditures as well as personnel time expenditure. When considering new techniques or equipment, examine precisely what will be needed by way of floor space, staffing, utilities, maintenance, service contracts, consumables, etc.

    Think about reimbursement levels. The key is to understand the hidden costs in ongoing operations that are not associated with the initial purchase. Identify the sources of reimbursement—direct patient billing, third-party and Medicare—before anticipating the next purchase. If it can't provide a return on investment, its purchase should be reconsidered.
- *Quality.* Not all benefits of new equipment are financial. Improvements in quality and productivity are less tangible but no less real. Will new equipment improve the quality of your department's services?

Planning to Acquire New Technologies

With the right information, strategic technology planning forms the basis for a coherent priority-setting and capital-budgeting process. Many hospitals rely on their medical staffs and financial planning departments to recommend and to determine the feasibility of acquiring new or replacement equipment. Instead, a technology assessment committee should oversee a capital equipment planning process that attends to the overall technology needs and strategic service goals of the hospital. How well this process works depends upon the talent, time, and resources of the individuals who have the task of researching and assessing new technology opportunities.

The initial step in technology planning is determining which new technologies deserve serious consideration and how they meet the strategic planning goals of the hospital.

Planning Considerations

The technology assessment process needs a mechanism in which the following planning tasks are accomplished.

1. **Monitoring**. Monitor and analyze the new and emerging technologies so that the development of new clinical services can be planned in advance. This requires the constant surveillance of diagnostic and therapeutic technologies.
2. **Assessing Impact**. Coordination with the organization's strategic plan, physician practice patterns and technology preferences, competition, staffing, space planning, physical and mechanical requirements and risks are all factors that have a significant impact on the decision-making process.
3. **Evaluating Costs**. Economic considerations (such as reimbursement, the effective life of the equipment, the expenses and revenues that will be generated and the decisions made by Medicare and other third-party payers about paying for new technology) must be carefully weighed in the planning process.

These planning considerations, when administered under an organized system of new technology assessment, set up a rational decision-making process that balances medical staff desires with hospital goals and financial restraints.

Technology Information Resources

For administrators who are looking for information about how technology may impact their facility, the following organizations are a valuable resource.

American Hospital Association
Division of Clinical Services and Technology
840 N. Lake Shore Drive
Chicago, IL 60611

American Medical Association
Diagnostic and Therapeutic Assessment
535 N. Dearborn Street
Chicago, IL 60610

Council on Health Care Technology
Institute of Medicine
2101 Constitution Avenue, NW
Washington, DC 20418

ECRI
5200 Bulter Pike
Plymouth Meeting, PA 19462

Johns Hopkins Program for Medical Technology and
    Practice Assessment
Center for Hospital Finance and Management
624 N. Broadway, Room 305
Baltimore, MD 21205

MD Buyline
5910 N. Central Expressway
Dallas, TX 75206

Medical Technology and Practice Patterns Institute
2233 Wisconsin Avenue NW, Suite 302
Washington, DC 20007

National Center for Health Services Research and
    Health Care Technology Assessment
Office of Health Technology Assessment
5600 Fishers Lane, Room 18A-27
Rockville, MD 20857

2.9   FUTURE TRENDS IN TECHNOLOGY

The world healthcare market was expected to spend $6 billion on diagnostic imaging equipment in 1992. Technology that was very experimental just a few years ago is now commonplace in radiology departments. New technologies from the broadcast and consumer electronics industries are being used to enhance medical imaging. Video processing and laser printers are just two of many examples of other technology making medical technology still better.

It was during the testing of supersonic jets in the 1960s that the evolution of lithotripsy was prompted. The impact of rain colliding with planes at supersonic speeds caused shock waves that damaged the aircraft even on the inside. What will come out of each new scientific discovery that has medical application cannot be predicted, but the prospects for an exciting future in the technology of medical imaging is assured.

Bone Densitometry

Clinical Indications

Osteoporosis is the most common metabolic disorder of the skeletal system. It is a serious loss of bone that results in crush fractures of the spine and fractures of the hip and wrist. Twenty million Americans are afflicted with the disease; 90 percent of whom are postmenopausal women. The diagnosis and treatment of this disorder costs approximately $6 billion per year.

The at-risk population for bone demineralization includes women with estrogen deficiency, recipients of long-time steroid therapy, primary asymptomatic hyperparathyroidism, end stage renal disease and vertebral anomalies. Risk factors for osteoporosis include age, weight, sex, height, cigarettes, alcohol, exercise, body frame, and calcium levels.

Bone densitometry has become an accepted tool for the diagnosis of osteoporosis. Increased experience with choosing the right measurement site and higher precision measuring devices has spurred a revolution of noninvasive bone mineral density assessment.

Technical Methods

Gone is the use of standard radiographs to measure bone density. Today, there are four noninvasive radiological methods commonly used for bone density assessment. These four major methods are well referenced for their clinical experience and are described here. Other modalities exist, but they are not widely used for clinical purposes.

Single-Photon Absorptiometry (SPA)

This modality has been in clinical use the longest. Approved for payment by HCFA in 1983, it remains the only bone densitometry technique reimburseable by Medicare. SPA has a high accuracy and precision, it is economical, and it uses negligible radiation dose. The measurement site is usually mid-shaft radius. A photon beam from a sealed 125 I radioisotope source is directed to the measurement site. The difference in photon absorption as measured by a detector opposite the beam source allows a calculation of bone mineral content.

Dual-Photon Absorptiometry (DPA)

As in the SPA device, there is a radioactive energy source and a detector. In the case of DPA, the radioactive energy source produces two photon energy peaks. Because the low energy photon beams are more attenuated in tissue than high energy photon beams, bone will produce a higher contrast between the two beams. This contrast difference is the operating principle of DPA. A highly automated report is prepared with computer-generated graphics.

Dual Energy Radiography (DER)

This technique is also known as quantitative digital radiography. The radioactive energy source is an x-ray tube that produces a two-peak energy spectrum. DER scanners allow high speed assessments with precision and low radiation dose. The DER devices have dominated sales of dedicated bone mass measurement devices since their introduction in 1987. Because the DER devices substitute x-ray for a radioactive source, an increase in photon flux occurs, which greatly improves scanning speed and spatial resolution.

Quantitative CT (QCT)

QCT was introduced commercially in 1984 and operates on a standard CT scanner modified with special software. The exam protocol for QCT involves scanning of three 1 cm thicknesses of trabecular bone in the lumbar spine. The radiation dose is much higher than with other techniques; x-ray exposure is up to 300 mrem as compared to 3 mrem with DER. QCT add-ons to existing CT scanners are a bargain at around $20,000, considerably less than a conventional bone densitometry system for $75,000 to $100,000.

Using a CT scanner to just measure bone mass, however, is not a very cost effective manner to utilize CT.

Discussion

The typical charge for an osteoporosis screening exam is $125 to $200. The clinical value of bone densitometry has sparked debate and slowed the development of this modality in the United States. The absence of federal reimbursement for dual photon techniques has influenced the position on coverage with other payers. About 40 percent of BC/BS carriers recognize bone densitometry as a reimbursable procedure; many private plans will cover the procedure. Making a positive bottom line in the reimbursement climate that exists today is difficult, especially for hospitals with their high fixed costs and overhead. Private physicians who control referrals can be moderately successful operating freestanding equipment in their offices. Gynecologists, rheumatologists, endocrinologists, nephrologists, and orthopedists will generate most of the referrals for this diagnosis. See figure 2.12 for industry over-view of current bone densitometry technology.

Magnetic Source Imaging (MSI)

As an emerging technology, the clinical usefulness of Magnetic Source Imaging has not been fully developed. When one considers that only 20 years ago many of the diagnostic technologies in use today were not available, the clinical promise of MSI is certainly a realistic proposition. In MSI, nerve impulses are propagated by the movement of ions that constitute electrical currents in neural tissues. Along with these currents are magnetic and electrical fields that come from the tissues and permeate the surrounding tissue strata. At this time, these fields are measured with familiar techniques such as electrocardiography and electroencephalography. Electrical fields are easily absorbed by bone, so detecting these fields using such devices positioned on the surface of the body suffer from the attenuation which occurs through bone. Magnetic fields are not as strongly attenuated by bone, therefore allowing their intensities to be mapped by superconducting quantum interference devices (SQUIDS). SQUIDS are very sensitive low noise amplifiers that pick up the

Figure 2.12   Who's Who In Bone Densitometry

Company Model	Price	Year Introduced	Number of Units
Single-Photon Absorptiometry			
Lunar			
SP2	$22,500	1985	130
Norland			
Norland-Cameron			
Bone Mineral Analyzer	$14,000	1970 (d)*	1500
Model 2780	$22,995	1980	n/a
Nuclear Data Systems			
ND1100	$28,500	1982	150
ND1100B	$19,500	1988	
Dual-Photon Absorptiometry			
Lunar			
DP3	$40,000	1981 (d 1988)	1120 (10% int'l)
Medical and Scientific Enterprises			
Osteotech	$50,000-$62,000	1988 (d 1989)	5
Polyscan 100	$70,000	1991	n/a
Norland			
2600	$39,995	1985 (d 1988)	n/a
Nuclear Data Systems			
ND2100	$35,000-$45,000	1982 (d 1989)	50
Single-Energy X-ray Absorptiometry			
Osteon			
Osteoanalyzer	$50,000	May 1991	160 (in US)
Dual-Energy X-ray Absorptiometry			
Hologic			
QDR-1000	$70,000	October 1987	750
QDR-1000/W	$80,000	December 1989	
QDR-2000	$100,000	November 1991	59
Lunar			
DPX	$55,000	June 1988	1035 (75% int'l)
DPX-L	$75,000	1990	(Reflects all DPX systems)
DPX-Alpha	$60,000	1990	
DPX-Plus	$60,000	1991	
DPX-Turbo	n/a	fall 1992	
Medical and Scientific Enterprises			
Polyscan 200	$80,000	pending FDA approval	–
Norland			
XR-26	$80,000	March 1989	n/a
XR-26 Mark II	$65,000	1991	n/a
Eclipse	$68,500	Sept. 1991	n/a

*(d) = discontinued

Figure 2.12 (Continued) Who's Who In Bone Densitometry

Company Model	Price	Year Introduced	Number of Units
Sopha Medical Systems			
Sophos L-XRA	n/a	pending FDA approval (1989 in Europe)	–
Ultrasound Bone Densitometry			
Lunar			
Achilles	$35,000	pending FDA approval (1991 in Europe)	–
Walker Sonix			
Ultrasonic Bone Analyzer	$25,000	pending FDA approval (1990 in Europe)	–
Quantitative Computed Tomography (QCT)			
Phantomless			
Columbia Scientific			
(share patient for phantomless QCT with IRIS)			
CSI/QCT	$10,000	1987	164
IM/QCT	$10,000	1991	5
Institute for Radiological Image Sciences (IRIS)			
(share patient for phantomless QCT with Columbia Scientific)			
PC/QCT	$10,000	1989	6
Phantom			
Computerized Imaging Reference Systems			
	company did not participate in survey		
GE Medical			
BMD	*company did not participate in survey*		
Image Analysis			
QCT-Bone Mineral Analysis	$17,400	1984	1,000
Philips			
(sells Image Analysis' QCT-Bone Mineral Analysis package with Philips software)	*company did not participate in survey*		
Siemens			
Osteo	*company did not participate in survey*		
Peripheral Quantitative Computed Tomography (pQCT)			
Norland			
XCT 900	$63,000	pending FDA approval	–

Source: published company data and *Second Source Imaging* estimates. Whelan, Mary C. Getting to the Bone. *Second Source Imaging.* 7(4): 50-57, 1992.

slightest amount of activity. The maps are used to compute the origin and strength of neural responses that created the measured magnetic fields. The neural events can be both spontaneous or responses to stimulus.

Clinical Applications

Initial clinical investigations suggest a scope of possible applications for MSI. In neurology, MSI can detect and locate brain tissues affected by stroke and TIA on the basis of abnormal electrical activity. The neurlogical application of MSI is especially exciting for the evaluation of patients with intractable epilepsy. MSI is also being explored as a method of evaluating migraine headache and diabetic coma.

In Cardiology, MSI may noninvasively locate the cause of arrhythmogenic tissue with enough accuracy for intervention with catheter ablation techniques. Also, MSI could provide a quantitative assessment of risk for the tendency to develop life threatening arrhythmias, help determine appropriate anti-arrhythmic drug therapy, and possibly monitor incipient rejection of transplanted hearts.

The Testing Procedure

At the Research Institute of Scripps Clinic in LaJolla, California, there is a 37-channel MSI system that represents the most sophisticated system in use today. A patient undergoing an MSI study is first demagnetized using a degausser wand. Because the system measures electrical activity, even minimal amounts of trace magnetism must be removed from the body. A special couch designed for securing the subject immovable for long periods of time is an important component of the system. The head is traced with another wand that allows the computer to simulate the shape and size of the skull. Devices are placed on the patient's fingers and lips and they deliver stimuli that is measured by the MSI system. The MSI sensor is a large cone-shaped device, which is placed over the subject's head. The entire procedure to scan the head takes approximately one hour. The computer-produced images of the brain portray the somatosensory and auditory cortices.

Infrared Imaging

Neurothermography, as it's called, is a technique that has been around since World War II. Similar to the humble beginnings of ultrasound with radar, early use of infrared in the military was for the nonvisible detection of enemy war machines. The use of thermography in medicine after the war has been a diagnostic modality that has come in and out of vogue. Recent advances in high resolution systems for imaging have caused renewed interest in medical infrared imaging.

How it Works

The largest organ of the body is the skin. It is a super heat regulator that continuously loses and preserves body heat with autonomic nervous control of blood flow to the external dermis layer of the skin. When there is a malfunction of a peripheral nerve's autonomic control, a correlating thermal asymmetry of the skin occurs. It is evidence of the thermal asymmetry that is documented with neurothermography. Very high definition equipment is available at a fairly high price. Infrared imaging packages with a selection of detector styles, computer, printer and archival methods are on the market for up to $100,000. It is a reimbursable imaging procedure and compares favorably in pricing with most ultrasound procedures. As a neuroimaging technique, it is an objective measure of autonomic nervous system abnormalities often encountered in the management of patients with chronic pain.

Angioplasty

In 1964, Dr. Charles Dotter performed the first documented angioplasty using a guidewire and a catheter. In 1970, Dr. W. Portsman developed the first balloon catheter. The double-lumen balloon catheter was introduced by Dr. Andreas Gruntzig in 1974. The basis of angioplasty is widening a narrowed area in an artery by pushing aside built up plaque deposits with an inflatable balloon. Restenosis rate with balloon angioplasty is fairly high, so instead of just dilating the artery, a method of cutting out the plaque called atherectomy can be used.

Percutaneous atherectomy devices can restore blood flow by cutting and removing atherosclerotic plaque. The technique is relatively safe, although danger of perforation to the arterial wall is a sometimes seen complication. The typical rotary atherectomy catheter uses a rotating cam to cut through atheroma tissue. Atherectomy technique is sometimes glibly referred to as "roto-rooter" of the arteries. Atherectomy can be performed alone or in conjunction with balloon angioplasty.

The objectives of various angioplasty techniques fall into three categories. Medically, the technique relieves symptoms and aids perfusion of the affected organ. The technical objective of angioplasty is to open a blocked area of the artery. The final objective is ease of application. It is a practical and economical alternative to surgery.

Categories of Angioplasty Devices

Dilatation is essentially pushing the plaque aside in the artery. It is done with tapered catheters, mechanical dilators, and balloons. Balloon angioplasty is one of the oldest methods of managing vascular obstructive disease and should continue to experience a good success rate.

Cutting devices (atherectomy) consist of augers, grinders, pulverizers, and shavers. The special catheters bore forward and remove the plaque in their path.

Stents work as a bridge or trussing to keep a dilated artery open. The stent forms an expandable frame for the artery to prevent restenosis. Two types of stents are currently being used: the self expandable and the balloon expanding stent. Key factors in the use of stents are ease of introduction, positioning, and ratio of unexpanded to expanded size.

Other techniques in use or under investigation are the disruption of plaque with ultrasound and dissolution of plaque with the controlled delivery of clot-specific thrombolytic drugs. Laser ablation may be accomplished with continuous and pulsed-wave lasers, contact probe, hot tip lasers, or indirect laser angioplasty. The use of lasers in the vascular system is a procedure that continues to be evaluated. Problems with restenosis rates and the safety of laser techniques has slowed the development of laser technology as a treatment and therapeutic modality for vascular disease.

Voice Recognition Technology

Producing written documents and distributing those reports is the present preoccupation of healthcare in general. The x-ray report is the permanent record of the interpretation of a radiologic examination. Whether it be the reported results of radiography, CT, ultrasound, MRI, or nuclear medicine, the "paper trail" is an endless source of frustration to managers and physicians. The JCAHO requires that the reports be timely. From a patient care point of view the quicker results reporting, the sooner medical management begins based on any findings. Legal and risk management requirements place additional pressure on results reporting. These records may end up in court and thus should be legible and complete.

The U.S. healthcare industry is very data intensive. Yet, this data-laden system is late to be computerized and automated. The bulk of documentation performed in healthcare today uses obsolete methods. Most medical record keeping is a manual process on paper that is stored in cramped filing areas. It is estimated that 80 percent of medical records are prose, and this prose is usually tape transcribed or handwritten.

The problems of generating the written radiology report and keeping track of those reports are well known to radiology managers. The solution may be the advent of voice recognition technology, a computer-based dictation system that allows direct transcription of words spoken into a phone. The radiologist speaks into an electronic device that recognizes words, displays them on a monitor, and prints a report. Voice recognition could make the human transcriptionist obsolete and imagine a typist who doesn't call in sick or request vacation time!

How it Works

When words dictated into the machine are compared with voice prints of words stored in the computer's memory, they are translated to the computer screen. The translations may be literal. The words appearing on the screen are exactly those spoken, or certain words may be used as "triggers" to prompt entire phrases to be displayed. (See Figure 2.13)

Figure 2.13   Voice Recognition Generated Report

Routine Mammography Report

SAY	DISPLAY
"today"	4/11/1990
"Prior exam 6/89"	Prior exam: 6/89
"mammography"	MAMMOGRAPHY: Bilateral
"bilateral"	
"routine"	A low dose film technique was used. Cephalocaudad and modified lateral views were obtained.
"slightly prominent nodules"	Both breasts show a slightly prominent duct pattern.
	There is diffuse nodularity, but there is no dominant mass or significant calcification.
"no facial lesions"	There are no dominant masses or clustered calcification on either side.
"obtain outside study"	We will attempt to obtain previous mammograms and an addendum will follow. If we do not obtain previous films re-examination in 6 months is recommended.
"signature"	John H. Jones, M.D. 9:18:32 4/11/1990

Reports like this can be generated in less than 30 seconds, using only 8 spoken words and phrases.

Courtesy of Kurzweil Applied Intelligence, Inc. Waltham, MA

The use of trigger words speeds up the dictation process by printing normal reports rapidly. Reports may also be constructed using "fill in the blank" techniques or the free text mode. Features of one manufacturer's equipment currently on the market include:

- Enables physicians to generate accurate patient records immediately, simply by speaking.
- Speaker adaptive—no user training needed, adapts to any accent.
- Functionally unlimited vocabulary allows physicians to generate a wide variety of patient reports.

- Trigger phrases enable physicians to call up report sections with a single spoken word.
- Can be integrated with hospital information systems to make reports instantly available.
- Edits reports by voice and prints simply by saying "print report."
- Supports the use of ICD-9 and CPT-4 billing and diagnosis codes to speed payment processing.
- System can be shared by several physicians, each with his or her own customized vocabulary.

More Technology Worth Monitoring

Slip ring technology allows for helical scanning in computed tomography (CT). The patient moves in a continuous fashion through the scanner and slices are acquired immediately following each other. In conventional CT the tube is prevented from continuous circling by its cables, thus a delay between each slice is needed for the tube to stop and reverse direction. Slip rings, grooved bands with a lining of electrically conductive brushes, take the place of cables. This helical scanning allows CT units to acquire volumetric data; it also will image moving organs with less misregistration.

Monoclonal antibodies (MABS) is a product of biotechnology. The monoclonal antibody is a guidance system for imaging agents. The MAB behaves like a microscopic bullet aimed at only one target, such as the antigen of a particular tumor. A MAB agent is used in nuclear imaging by mixing the antibody with a radioisotope such as indium or technetium. The MAB tagged radioisotope is injected into the patient and the antibodies move through the bloodstream looking for their target. Once the MABs bind to their target (e.g., a malignant lesion in the colon), imaging then takes place with a nuclear camera. MAB imaging techniques are mainly divided between oncology and cardiac applications. In cardiac imaging, MABs connect with dead heart tissue and show the extent of damage following heart attack.

Electric Impedance Imaging (EII), Microwave Computed Tomography, Visible Light Imaging (transillumination), **3D Ultrasound, Nonclaustrophobic MRI, Twin CT, Image Distribution Systems** and **Dry Process Laser Film** printing are just a few innovations in a list of new technological developments. Today, there is a flourish of technological development in medical imaging. Some of this new technology will become important in the day-to-day practice of radiology; some may need much more development before it has immediate practical significant impact on patient care.

2.10 FINANCING NEW TECHNOLOGY

Hospitals are facing many threats to their ability to generate a positive margin on daily operations. Financing equipment acquisitions in a cash crunch environment places administrators in a position in which they must be very selective about the equipment they buy. The decision to buy is based on a large part on the equipment's ability to generate profits. See Figure 2.14.

The financial feasibility study for the acquisition of new technology needs to investigate those variables that will directly influence the generation of gross revenue. These variables, when combined, must produce a sufficient revenue stream to cover the operating costs of the equipment.

Figure 2.14 Profitable Healthcare Equipment (Listed in Rank Order)

CT Scanners
Automated Lab Equipment
R and F Rooms
Spect Cameras
Ultrasound
Cardiac Cath Labs
Nuclear Medicine
Mammography
Heart Lung Machines
MRI
Mobile Cardiac Cath
Radiation Therapy
Lasers
PET
Mobile Lithotripsy
Mobile Cardiac Cath
Lithotripters
Patient Monitoring
Ambulances
Helicopters

Adapted from American Hospital Publishing and the Linc Group, Inc. 1990.

Revenue Variables

The purpose of a financial analysis is to investigate a set of variables and assumptions and develop a model that will estimate increased revenues earned and the additional expenditures that result (in this instance) from the acquisition of a new piece of equipment. These include:

* Demand.
* Volume.
* Time.
* Charge.
* Reimbursement.

Market demand is the first and most important variable to help determine whether opportunity for increased revenues exists. In the case of new technology, market demand is dictated by the level of procedure **volume** that the proposed new service will generate. When analyzing demand (1) quantify the number of units of service, (2) determine the **time** it takes to complete a procedure, and (3) investigate if identical equipment exists elsewhere and whether its rate of utilization meets the current demand for the service. When the volume of procedures has been predicted, the **charge** per unit of service is then established based on what is reasonable and necessary to produce at least a break-even financial scenario. When establishing charges, it is imperative that each third party payer be investigated in respect to **reimbursement**. The mix of payers is a very important consideration in making assumptions about revenue variables. A high percentage of Medicare reimbursement, for instance, may have an adverse effect on predicting profitability of a new service. A demand analysis combined with a charge analysis is a key factor in determining the net income potential of the new service.

Expenses

An analysis of costs is the other side of the equation when attempting to accurately project net cash flow that can result from new technology. When developing a proforma to justify the acquisition of a new piece of equipment, the analysis should address fixed and variable costs as well as indirect and direct expenses. Keep in mind that it will be the variable costs that will be most difficult to accurately quantify. The variable costs are expenditures that will fluctuate with service volumes. Consider the answers to the following questions that address issues related to expense variables.

- What will be the direct/fixed cost of purchasing the equipment?
- What will be the direct/fixed cost of renovation or construction?
- What will it cost to finance or lease the equipment?
- What will personnel expenses be?
- Will there be service expenses directly related to the new equipment (i.e., maintenance contracts, insurance policies)?
- What will the expenses of administrative support entail (i.e., billing, accounting, office supplies)?
- What variable costs are associated with providing the new service (i.e., supplies, utilities)? (See Figure 2.15)

Figure 2.15 Proforma Mobile Mammography

Patient Volume				
# of patients per day	12	18	22	25
# of patients per month @ 22 days/mo.	264	396	484	550
Gross Revenue per Month				
Patients per mo. @ $65 ea.	$17,160	$25,740	$31,460	$35,750
Variable Costs				
Reading Fee @ $15 per patient	$3,960	$5,940	$7,260	$8,250
Utilization Costs @ $7.50 per patient	$1,980	$2,970	$3,630	$4,125
Net Revenue				
Per Month	$11,220	$16,830	$20,570	$23,375
Fixed Monthly Expenses				
Van Lease	$4,200	$4,200	$4,200	$4,200
Salaries				
2 Techs @ $22,000/yr.	$4,877	$4,877	$4,877	$4,877
.5 Manager @ $30,000/yr	$1,633	$1,633	$1,633	$1,633
Miscellaneous Overhead	$1,000	$1,000	$1,000	$1,000
Total Monthly Expenses				
Fixed	$11,739	$11,739	$11,739	$11,739
Monthly Net Profit or				
(Loss)	($519)	$5,091	$8,831	$11,636
Annual Profit or (Loss)	($6,230)	$61,090	$105,970	$139,630

Adapted from "On the Road: Planning and Operating a Mobile Mammography Program" by Patricia Courson. *Administrative Radiology.* 10(4): 48-58, 1991.

Buy or Lease

Leasing can be an attractive financing option for equipment that is evolving rapidly. Technological obsolescence and no down payment are cited as frequent advantages to lease plans. There are a number of reasons to consider a lease arrangement to acquire new technology. These reasons are very unique to the healthcare industry. A better understanding of leasing versus buying can yield substantial financial dividends.

- A cash outlay is made more difficult because of the risks involved with increased competition, a shrinking reimbursement environment, and increased costs of operations.
- The capital pass-through reimbursement with Medicare is available when leasing equipment.
- Less tax exempt financing and declining hospital bond ratings have made borrowing money more difficult.
- More debt financing is not an option for already overburdened hospital balance sheets.

Leasing Options

The selection of an equipment lessor should depend on a total program approach. The total program approach will include residual values, purchase and renewal options, lease term, and other costs such as taxes and shipping expenses.

The leasing industry uses a variety of terms to characterize leases: true lease, leveraged lease, lease-purchase, conditional sale, operating lease, full payout, and tax oriented. Obviously, when selecting a financial instrument and evaluating a leasing agent, a thorough understanding of the leasing industry is a prerequisite negotiation tool.

Leasing is an option worth considering when the equipment has a high likelihood of obsolescence or cash flow is a problem. Today, there are numerous reputable equipment lessors that provide a wide variety of lease financing products. Knowledge of the leasing process is the best defense for choosing the lease plan that will meet your needs with the most favorable terms.

Additional Strategies for Meeting the Costs of New Technology

* Coordinate interests with physicians and other institutions, develop joint ventures, and plan to minimize duplicate service.
* Consider a partnership with a manufacturer in exchange for research and development of a particular new technology.
* Become a demonstration site for manufacturers in exchange for a more attractive purchase price.
* Establish a training program to make human resources available to support and operate new technology.

Conclusion

The trends affecting healthcare technology development (competition, quality, cost-containment, legislation, and social demographics) have become a constant and are not likely to change much in the years to come. There are few rivals to the healthcare industry for dependence upon technology. Successful providers of the future will need to creatively analyze emerging technologies, identify those opportunities for profit, and find the financing plans needed to assure market position.

2.11 MRI—FEASIBILITY OF A NEW SERVICE

How do you begin to determine whether the purchase of MR technology is a good decision for your organization? According to *Healthweek*, there were nearly 2,000 installed units in the United States as of December 1990. (See Figure 2.16) It is quite understandable for a radiologist to want access to MRI; it is now impossible to practice modern diagnostic radiology without it. Professional medical literature is filled with references to the clinical efficacy of MRI in diagnosis for neurology, neurosurgery, and orthopedics. A good place to begin your MRI feasibility study is with the creation of a business plan.

Figure 2.16 Magnetic Resonance Imagers

Company	Total MRI Installed
GE Medical System	849
Siemens Medical Systems, Inc.	323
Toshiba America Medical Systems, Inc.	265
Picker International, Inc.	205
Fonar Corp.	130
Phillips Medical Systems North America Co.	106
Resonex, Inc.	40
Elscint, Inc.	30
Hitachi American, Ltd.	22
Instrumentarium Imaging, Inc.	14
Shimadzu Medical Systems	6
Burker Medical Imaging, Inc.	6
Total	1996

Source: *Healthweek.* November, 1990.

The Business Plan

A business plan is a management tool; it helps to focus in a logical and organized fashion the direction your project will take. The business plan is also a control tool that allows you to monitor and to evaluate the progress of your program. Elements of a good business plan include: a business description, market analysis, a service/ product description, market strategy, an operations overview, management and organization, timing and a financial analysis. (A business plan will be examined in greater detail elsewhere in this text).

Predicting Utilization

The American Hospital Association Demand Forecast Model for MRI utilization offers three different predictions of MRI scan volume. One is an ICD-9-CM projection method and two use DRG information. Study your hospital or clinic's DRG and ICD-9 profiles. Look closely at current utilization of all imaging modalities. It is possible that up to 40 percent of procedures that you are currently performing are reimbursable as MR procedures.

Generally, the use of MRI has been directed towards only a few clinical applications. Increased use of MRI in the extremities, the recent introduction of more contrast agents, and the potential for MR angiography suggests that the national forecast for scans may reach 6.4 million per year. This scanning volume will increase the installed base of MRI units to over 3,000 during the decade of the 1990s. Also, during the next decade, low cost specialty units will be found in the smallest hospitals and clinics. These new units will be easy to site and scan faster. The benefits of MR as a noninvasive diagnostic technique without the use of radiation will encourage increased use and new clinical applications. Possibly, the use of MRI as a diagnostic modality will overtake CT in hospitals.

Determining MR Needs

Before committing to an important investment like MRI, there will be many questions to answer in order to determine your exact MR needs. The major question is whether your hospital or clinic can support an MR system. This is a critical factor because patient volume will drive the financial feasibility of the project. Predicting volume may be greatly assisted by using an American Hospital Association Demand Forecast Model. Another important consideration is assessing your current referral base. Most of your patients will be referred by physicians and clinics in your service area. It will be important to segment your referring physicians by speciality, since referral volume in an MRI service varies considerably from specialist to specialist. Adding an MRI service to your hospital or clinic may actually attract physicians to your area. Because referring physicians are the primary source for MR business, understanding your current physician base and determining what new specialties you may attract may have some bearing on some specific system features of your MRI service.

The overall market picture in your service area will dictate your procedure and referral potential. It will be necessary for you to understand the population mix of the area that you wish to serve. If there is a high concentration of physicians with a particular specialty in your area, you will want to anticipate their demands on your MR facility. Key components of a market assessment will include: definition of the service area, demographic survey of the population, analysis of the competition, and analysis of the referring physician base.

Finally, understand your current payor mix. Did the demographic assessment of the population in your service area suggest that a high percentage of your patients will be private insurance? If you must rely on Medicare reimbursement rather than on third-party payors, what will the effect be on your balance sheet?

The Financial Picture

According to Howard W. Schwartz, senior administrative director of radiology at the University of Minnesota Hospital and Clinic, a realistic proforma analysis should support a capital investment such as MRI. Assuming the need for MRI meets tests of appropriateness, efficacy, and marketability, it still needs to be a financially sound scenario. The analysis should include an accurate projection of expected volume and pricing, with contractual allowances that will produce a net revenue that pays the project expenses in a reasonable time frame. Payback should occur within the useful life of the scanner. (See Figure 2.17) Common error and omissions in financial proformas to avoid include: overestimated revenues, underestimated expenses, poorly defined assumptions, and poor predictions of contractual allowances.

Figure 2.17 MRI Financial Feasibility

Purchase Price	$2,500,000
Useful Life	5 years
Depreciation	$500,000
Construction/Renovation	$1,500,000
Useful Life	10 years
Annual Depreciation	$150,000
Projected Revenue **(1)**	$2,200,000
Projected Expenses **(2)**	$1,200,000
Return on Investment **(3)**	1.6 years

(1) 2,000 exams at $1400 each, 21% contractual adjustments yield a total net revenue of $2,200,000.

(2)	Salaries	$100,000
	Maintenance	250,000
	Depreciation	650,000
	Supplies	100,000
	Interest Income	100,000
		$1,200,000

(3) Purchase price divided by (Revenue - Expenses + Depreciation)

Adapted from Schwartz, H.W. "Justifying Capital Equipment in the 1990's." *Radiology Management*. 12(2):35-39, 1990.

Appendix A

*Directory of Technologist Education in MRI**

Arizona

Saint Joseph's Hospital and Medical Center
Radiologic Education Center
350 West Thomas Rd.
Phoenix, AZ 85013-4496
(602) 285-3956 or (602) 285-3957
Length: one week

California

Loma Linda University
Department of Radiologic Technology,
School of Allied Health Professions
Loma Linda, CA 92350
(800) 422-4558 or (714) 824-4931
Length: six months

Toshiba America MRI Inc.
Clinical Education Department
280 Utah Ave.
South San Francisco, CA 94080
(415) 872-2722
Length: one week

Delaware

Delaware Technical Community College,
Southern Campus
Department of Radiology
P.O. Box 610
Georgetown, DE 19947
(302) 856-5400, ext. 517
Length: two months

District of Columbia

George Washington University Medical Center
Radiologic Sciences and Administration Program
Radiologic Allied Health Office, Room 616
2300 I St., NW
Washington, DC 20037
(202) 994-3650
Length: four or eight months

Florida
Furon Training Center, Advanced Medical
Diagnostics/MRI Center
    442 Fourth Ave.
    Indialantic, FL 32903
    (800) 473-0855 or (407) 728-0855
    Length: one week
Georgia
Emory University Hospital
    School of Radiologic Technology
    1364 Clifton Road, NE
    Atlanta, GA 30322
    (404) 727-6133
    Length: four months
Emory University Hospital
    Magnetic Resonance Education Center
    Atlanta, GA 30322
    (404) 727-5864
    Length: one week
Idaho
Boise State University
    Department of Radiographic Science
    1910 University Drive
    Boise, ID 83725
    (208) 385-1996
    Length: eight months
Iowa
The University of Iowa Hospitals and Clinics
    C-723 Radiology
    Iowa City, IA 52242
    (319) 356-4332
    Length: six months
Maryland
Johns Hopkins Hospital
    Department of Radiology
    Program in Advanced Imaging
    601 North Wolfe St.
    Baltimore, MD 21205
    (301) 955-5510
    Length: 12 months

New Jersey

Medical Imaging Consultants, Inc.
2227 U.S. Hwy. 1, Suite 225
North Brunswick, NJ 08902
(908) 745-2310
Length: three days

New York

MR Imaging
4273 Hempstead Turnpike
Bethpage, NY 11714
(516) 579-5800
Length: one or two weeks

Long Island University, CW Post Campus
Department of Health Professions
Northern Blvd.
Brookeville, NY 11548
(516) 299-3075
Length: two or three months

Fonar Corporation, Training Department
110 Marcus Drive
Melville, NY 11747
(516) 694-2929
Length: one week

Ohio

The Kettering College of Medical Arts
Department of Imaging Sciences
3737 Southern Blvd.
Kettering, OH 45429
(800) 296-5262 or (513) 296-7201, ext. 5696
Length: four months

The Ohio State University
Magnetic Resonance Imaging Facility
1630 Upham Drive
Columbus, OH 43210
(614) 293-5172
Length: one week

Pennsylvania

Hospital of The University of Pennsylvania
Department of Radiology/MRI Continuing Education
3400 Spruce St., 1 Founders Building

Philadelphia, PA 19104
(215) 662-6877
Length: one week
The University of Pittsburgh
Department of Radiology/NMR Institute of Pittsburgh
3260 Fifth Ave.
Pittsburgh, PA 15213
(412) 647-6674
Length: three weeks

Tennessee
Chattanooga State Technical Community College
Department of Allied Health, MRI Program
4501 Amnicola Highway
Chatttanooga, TN 37406
(615) 697-4450
Length: four months

Texas
Advanced Health Education Center
102 Portland
Houston, TX 77006
(713) 522-8702
Length: four weeks
The University of Texas Southwestern Medical Center
Department of Radiology
5323 Harry Hines Road
Dallas, TX 75235-8896
(214) 688-8013
Length: one or four weeks
The University of Texas Medical Brunch
School of Allied Health Sciences
Radiologic Health Sciences/Health-Related Sciences
Internal Mail Route #J-28
Galveston, TX 77550
(409) 761-3042
Length: four months

Utah
Weber State University
MRI Program
Ogden, UT 84408-1602
(801) 626-7156
Length: 12 months

Virginia
  The University of Virginia Health Sciences Center
    Department of Radiology, Medical Imaging Division
    P.O. Box 486
    Charlottesville, VA 22908
    (804) 924-9384
    Length: 12 months
Wisconsin
  MTMI
    P.O. Box 26337
    Milwaukee, WI 53226
    (800) 765-6864 or (414) 774-2233
    Length: one or two weeks

---

* List prepared by C.J. Skillington for *R.T. Image Magazine*. Oct. 26, 1992.

2.12 MRI PURCHASE CONSIDERATIONS

The MR decision requires careful consideration, planning, and consensus building because the investment in this high technology radiology equipment is substantial. How can the perspective buyer negotiate multiple factors such as financial, medical, and marketing that impact the selection process? The MR decision is influenced by many considerations, including the following:

- How to evaluate the MR Imagers in the product literature and trade shows.
- Which equipment features are critical to future development and new applications?
- Which equipment features influence patient throughput?
- What to look at and which questions to ask during a site visit.
- What will be the service arrangement?
- What training is available for physicians and technologists?
- Other than system price, what factors impact financial risk?

General Electric Medical Systems has published a "Buyers' Guide to Evaluating MR Systems." It is a concise guide for anyone involved in the MR purchase decision. It is available from General Electric free of charge. Another GE publication, "Administrators' Guide to MR," is also available free of charge and contains very helpful information.

What to Look for in a System and Manufacturer*

Image Quality

Image quality should be considered within the context of time (how long it took and is it a realistic scan time?) and of diagnostic relevance. The ability to produce high quality images under exacting parameters is key to a good system. Also, high quality imaging depends on optimal performance of critical system features. Consider:

- A broad range of fields of view.
- A broad range of slice thicknesses, without field of view restrictions.
- T_1 weighted images with echo times less than 30 milliseconds routinely and capability for 20 milliseconds.
- T_2 weighted images—especially body images—that combine thin slices, small fields of view, high resolution matrices, and short acquisition times.
- Overall image uniformity with no loss of edge definition.
- High magnetic field homogeneity.
- High radio frequency field homogeneity.
- Motion compensation software.
- High field strength.

Clinical Flexibility

The ability to perform a broad range of applications increases referrals. The greater the system's adaptability to new techniques, the longer the useful life of the capital investment. Consider:

- Multi-slice, multi-angle oblique imaging in any plane.
- T_1 and T_2 weighted images with small fields of view and thin slices.
- Ability to scan in high resolution matrix with single excitation.
- Exacting imaging parameters with a reasonable scan time.
- High speed, linear gradience.

---

*Adapted from "Buyers' Guide to Evaluating MR Systems." GE Medical Systems. 1986. Used with permission.

- Powerful, flexible control module that's easily programmed.
- High data transfer rates.
- Eddy current compensation.
- Image processing with sufficient memory and flexibility.

Productivity

Enhanced operating efficiency and department productivity are more considerations:

- Simple operator/system interface.
- Efficient filming and archiving.
- Fast data reconstruction.
- Patient friendly features (e.g., lighted, well-ventilated tunnel).
- 95 percent or higher patient acceptance rate.
- Mobile patient transport.

Siting and Service Programs

Siting assistance from the manufacturer is an important consideration in the MR decision process. A well-planned installation will save mistakes that will jeopardize future system performance. Service has a significant impact on the day-to-day performance of an MR system. Consider:

- A proven track record.
- Layout schematics.
- Evaluation of alternative sites.
- Instrumentation study of each site.
- Complete magnetic shielding analysis and design, and proven magnetic shielding experience.
- Protection against magnet/cryostat damage, including replacement of the magnet.
- On-call and remedial service.
- Well-stocked local parts source plus round-the-clock access to parts network.
- Prompt response time.
- A comprehensive program: cryogens and equipment maintenance/repair.
- Point-by-point explanation of the program(s).
- Planned maintenance and system recalibration.

- Option of second or third shift maintenance.
- Complete cryogen service, with a fixed price for cryogens.

Other Considerations

The site visit is another important part of the MR evaluation process. You will see a system in clinical use and talk to the professionals that use the equipment every day. Most importantly, you will see images produced under true clinical conditions. Be prepared to ask lots of questions and test the manufacturer's claims of performance.

Figure 3.4   Sample floor plan of a compact but efficient MRI facility

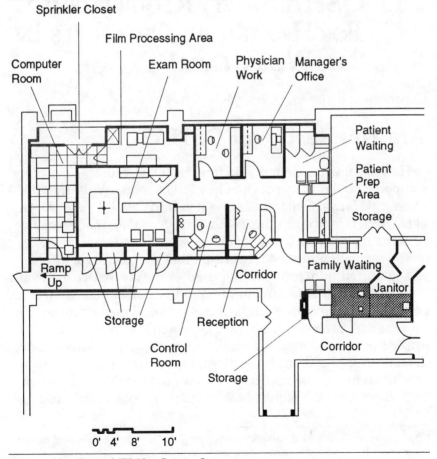

Sprinkler Closet

Film Processing Area

Computer Room

Exam Room

Physician Work

Manager's Office

Patient Waiting

Patient Prep Area

Storage

Ramp Up

Corridor

Family Waiting

Janitor

Storage

Reception

Control Room

Storage

Corridor

0' 4' 8'   10'

Courtesy New Britain MRI. New Britain, Conn.

Also, check to see that a program is in place for future development that is backed with strong clinical research. What will be the risk of obsolescence with the system? Look for manufacturers that minimize the necessity for forklift upgrades and that will demonstrate quick payback on other system upgrades as they become available. Seek a company with a strong strategic plan for future growth and clinical development.

Finally, investigate the manufacturer to be assured that long-term financial stability exists.

2.13 OSHA SAFETY REQUIREMENTS FOR HAZARDOUS CHEMICALS IN THE WORKPLACE*

Contributed by James Dohms, B.S., R.T.

Are You Ready for OSHA?

How would your department fare if an OSHA compliance officer stopped by today to inspect for chemical hazards? While the OSHA Chemical Hazard Communication Standard (29 CFR 1910.1200) has been in effect for the healthcare industry since 1987, many radiology administrators are unaware of all the standard's requirements.

The regulation's intent is to ensure that the hazards of all chemicals imported into, produced, or used in the workplace are evaluated, and that this hazard information is transmitted to affected employers and exposed employees. Chemical manufacturers and importers must convey the hazard information they learn from their evaluations to downstream employers by issuing a material safety data sheet, or MSDS, and by putting labels on containers. All covered employers must have a program to communicate this information to their employees through container labeling, MSDSs and training.

---

*This article on hazardous communication appeared in the Fall, 1992 issue of *Radiology Management*. It is reprinted here with the permission of the author.

Radiology administrators must become familiar with the standard so they can fulfill its requirements. The following details of the standard deserve special attention.

Compiling a List of Hazardous Chemicals

The first step in implementing a hazard communication program is to complete a thorough inventory of all chemicals found in the department. This includes chemicals such as disinfectants, fixer, developer and certain instrument cleaners. You may not know which products in the department are hazardous until you receive and review the material safety data sheet for that product.

OSHA exempts any consumer product or hazardous substance that is shown to be used in the workplace the same way it is used by normal consumers, and for a duration and frequency of exposure that is not greater than that experienced by consumers. For example, if dishwashing detergent is occasionally used to clean dishes in the imaging facility, it would be exempted from the standard's requirements as long as the quantity of detergent in the facility is not greater than that normally found in the home. However, using bleach to disinfect imaging equipment would not be considered normal consumer use and would fall under the requirements.

Foods, drugs or cosmetics intended for personal consumption by employees at work are exempted from the standard. Any drug—as defined in the Federal Food, Drug, and Cosmetic Act (21 U.S.C. 301 *et seq.*)—that is in final form for direct administration to the patient (i.e., tablets or pills) is also exempt from the standard. The key phrase of that exemption is "final form." Therefore, contrast agents and drugs in cream or liquid form fall under the requirements of the standard.

Once you have compiled a complete list of potentially hazardous chemicals, the next step is to compare the list with the material safety data sheets you may already have on hand. For any MSDSs that are missing, contact your supplier and request one. It is important to document these requests in the event OSHA reviews your hazard communication program before you receive the missing MSDS.

Having a Written Program

All workplaces where employees are exposed to hazardous chemicals must have a written hazard communication program, which describes how the department plans to meet the requirements for labels and other forms of warning, material safety data sheets, and employee information and training. Paragraph "e" of the standard spells out the specific requirements. The written program need not be lengthy or complicated (see sample program at the end of this article). If an OSHA compliance officer inspects your facility, he or she will ask to see the program at the beginning of the inspection process. Failure to provide a written program will result in a citation.

Labeling Containers

The OSHA standard requires that each container of hazardous chemical in the workplace be labeled, tagged or marked with the following information:

—The name and address of the chemical's manufacturer or other responsible party;
—The identity of the hazardous chemical(s) contained therein; and
—The appropriate hazard warnings, which can be any type of message, words, pictures, or symbols that convey the hazards of the chemical(s) in the container.

An exception to the labeling requirement is when hazardous chemicals are transferred from labeled containers and are intended only for the immediate use of the employee who performs the transfer.

In the medical setting, employees commonly use spray bottles containing disinfectants, trays filled with sterilizing solutions, and containers used along with bulk liquids, such as isopropyl alcohol. Often, radiology facilities fail to meet certain requirements of the standard because containers are not labeled properly. For example, OSHA fined one hospital in the Midwest for having an unlabeled container of a ten percent mixture of bleach and water. The point is, radiology administrators can easily comply with the labeling requirement by attaching the appropriate information on unlabeled containers.

Material Safety Data Sheets

The chemical manufacturer or distributor must automatically provide the end user with a material safety data sheet (MSDS) for all hazardous chemicals. That data sheet must be provided at the time of initial shipment and with the first shipment after a material safety data sheet is updated. Under the rule, there is no specified format for the MSDS, although there are specific information requirements. The purpose of the MSDS is to provide information on each hazardous chemical—its chemical and physical properties, the hazards associated with the chemical and the recommended protective measures that should be followed. The radiology administrator should be primarily concerned with the information on hazardous effects and recommended protective measures.

Material safety data sheets must be readily accessible to employees when they are in their work areas. In the radiology facility, using a binder in the control area is acceptable, whereas keeping the MSDSs in an office that is sometimes locked does not satisfy the intent of the standard.

Informing and Training Employees

One of the most important aspects of the Hazard Communication Standard is providing employees with information and training on hazardous chemicals in their work area. That training must take place prior to assigning an employee to work with a hazardous chemical, and whenever the hazard changes. Employees must be informed of:

- The provisions of the Hazard Communication Standard;
- Any operations in employees' work areas where hazardous chemicals are present;
- The location and availability of the department's written hazard communication program, including mandatory list(s) of hazardous chemicals and MSDSs required by the Hazard Communication Standard;
- Methods and observations that may be used to detect the presence or release of a hazardous chemical in the work area;
- Measures employees can take to protect themselves from these hazards, including information on work practices, emergency procedures and personnel protective equipment required by the employer; and
- Details of the employer's written hazard communication program, including an explanation of the labeling system used by the employer, MSDSs, and how employees can obtain and use the appropriate hazard information on the labels and in the MSDSs.

Employers may provide information and training by individual chemical or by hazard categories (such as corrosive materials or flammable liquids). As part of the inspection process, OSHA compliance officers will speak with employees to determine (a) if they are aware that they are exposed to hazardous chemicals, (b) if they know how to read and use the information found on material safety data sheets and labels, (c) whether they have received training, and (d) if they are following appropriate protective measures. According to OSHA publicaton 3111, "Hazard Communication Guidelines for Compliance," "OSHA does not expect that every worker will be able to recite all the information about each chemical in the workplace." Nevertheless, employees who are well informed about the chemical hazards found in the workplace are more likely to follow the proper precautions for reducing the chances of a serious accident.

Compliance in Radiology

Radiology administrators should pay special attention to the chemical hazards that are inherent in their imaging facilities. For example, the chemicals that make up developer and fixer are corrosive and should be handled with caution. (Here the term "corrosive" is defined as the effects of a substance on the eyes or skin, not surfaces.) Is it a policy in your facility to require personnel who replenish premixed chemistry to wear protective eyewear when doing so? Do you have an eyewash that is readily available in the event of an exposure incident? If the answer is no to either of these questions, your facility may be faced with an OSHA citation or a liability suit if an incident occurs.

The use of temporary personnel in the radiology facility is commonplace. Radiology administrators must ensure that, before these personnel are assigned to tasks exposing them to hazardous chemicals, they receive information and training that is specific to each facility. Topics that are unique and should be covered include the location of material safety data sheets, operations in the work area where hazardous chemicals are present, and the procedures implemented to protect employees in the facility, including the availability and required use of personal protective equipment. Radiology administrators should also repeat specific chemical training sessions as required by the standard since the level of training will vary among temporary personnel.

The standard does not apply to office workers if they encounter hazardous chemicals only in isolated instances. OSHA considers most office products (such as pens, pencils, adhesive tape) to be exempt under the provisions of the rule. Correction fluid such as Liquid Paper is also exempt as long as it is packaged in the same form and concentration as those intended for use by the general public. Intermittent or occasional use of a copying machine does not fall under the rule, although employees who handle the chemicals to service the machine, or operate it for long periods of time, are subject to the requirements of the Hazard Communication Standard.

Other Requirements and Regulations

Employees may be asked to perform nonroutine tasks that expose them to hazardous chemicals. OSHA requires that employees be provided with training before they undertake these tasks.

The OSHA Hazard Communication Standard does not require employers to maintain records of employee training, though many employers choose to do so.

Many states have additional regulations, sometimes referred to as Right-to-Know Laws, covering hazardous substances in the workplace. These regulations may require annual employee training, documentation of training, contain specific training requirements, or require the maintenance of MSDSs for chemicals no longer used in the facility, for a specified number of years.

Additional Information

OSHA has published a number of pamphlets designed to assist employers in developing a hazard communication plan. You can obtain these pamphlets from your local OSHA office or by writing to the Superintendent of Documents, Government Printing Office, Washington, D.C. 20402. Ordering information: *Chemical Hazard Communication*, OSHA 3084; *Hazard Communication Guidelines for Compliance*, OSHA 3111; *Hazard Communication, A Compliance Kit*, OSHA 3104 ($18.00, GPO order number 929-022-00000-9)

Bibliography

U.S Department of Labor, Occupational Safety and Health Administration. *Hazard Communication Guidelines for Compliance.* OSHA 3111, 1991, pp. 5-15.

U.S. Department of Labor, Occupational Safety and Health Administration. *Hazard Communication Standard.* 29 CFR Ch XVII (7-1-91 Edition), pp. 351-367.

U.S. Department of Labor, Occupational Safety and Health Administration. *Hazard Communication Guidelines for Compliance.* OSHA 3104, 1988, pp. J1-J3.

Sample Hazard Communication Program

General Department Policy

The purpose of this notice is to inform you that our hospital radiology department is complying with the OSHA Hazard Communication Standard, Title 29 Code of Federal Regulations 1910.1200, by (a) compiling a hazardous chemicals list, (b) using material safety data sheets (MSDSs), (c) ensuring that containers are labeled, and (d) providing you with training.

This program applies to all work operations in the radiology department where you may be exposed to hazardous substances under normal working conditions or during an emergency situation.

The radiology safety officer, Lois Smith, is the program coordinator, acting as the representative of the radiology director, who has overall responsibility for the program. Ms. Smith will review and update the program, as necessary. Copies of the written program may be obtained from her in Room A-5.

Under this program, you will be informed of the contents of the Hazard Communication Standard, the hazardous properties of chemicals with which you work, safe handling procedures, and measures to take to protect yourself and others from these chemicals. You will also be informed of the hazards associated with nonroutine tasks such as replenishing premixed processor chemistry tanks or removing processor racks in the event of a film jam.

List of Hazardous Chemicals

The safety officer will make a list of all hazardous chemicals and related work practices used in the department, and will update the list as necessary. Our list identifies all the chemicals that are used in this department. A copy of the list can be found on the pages preceding this policy and also serves as an index for the book of MSDSs which is maintained in the control area.

Material Safety Data Sheets (MSDSs)

MSDSs provide you with specific information on the chemicals you use. The safety officer, Ms. Smith, will maintain a binder in the control area of the radiology department. An MSDS on every substance found on the list can be found in the binder. The MSDS will be a fully completed OSHA Form 174 or equivalent. The safety officer is responsible for acquiring and updating MSDSs. She will contact the chemical manufacturer or vendor if additional research is necessary or if an MSDS has not been supplied with an initial shipment. All new procurements for the radiology department must be cleared by the safety officer.

Labels and Other Forms of Warning

The radiology safety officer will ensure that all hazardous chemicals in the radiology department are properly labeled and updated, as necessary. Labels should at least list the chemical identity, appropriate hazard warnings, and the name and address of the manufacturer, importer or other responsible party. Ms. Smith will refer to the corresponding MSDS to assist you in verifying label information.

Contrast agents, both oral and injectable, and other drugs found in the radiology department are exempt from the container labeling requirements. Refer to the appropriate MSDS if you have questions concerning the safe handling and appropriate protective measures you should take when working with these substances.

If you transfer chemicals from a labeled container to a portable container that is intended for your immediate use, no labels are required on the portable container. The transfer of chemicals from a labeled container into a portable container that will be used by others beside yourself and for nonimmediate use must be labeled. If you have questions regarding this requirement, contact your immediate supervisor or the safety officer, Ms. Smith, before making the transfer.

Nonroutine Tasks (Technologists and Darkroom Personnel)

In order to prepare you to perform hazardous nonroutine tasks (e.g, replenishing premixed processor chemistry tanks or removing processor racks in the event of a film jam), a special training session will be conducted to inform you about the hazardous chemicals to which you might be exposed and the proper precautions to take to reduce or avoid exposure.

Training

Everyone who works with, or is potentially exposed to, hazardous chemicals will receive initial training on the Hazard Communication Standard and the safe use of those hazardous chemicals by the radiology safety officer. A program that uses both audiovisual materials and classroom-type training has been prepared for this purpose. Whenever a new hazardous chemical is introduced into the radiology department, additional training will be provided. Supervisors will be extensively trained on hazards and appropriate protective measures so they will be available to answer questions from employees and provide daily monitoring of safe work practices.

The training program will emphasize these items:

- Summary of the standard and this written program;
- Chemical and physical properties of hazardous materials (e.g., reactivity, volatility) and methods that can be used to detect the presence or release of chemicals;
- Health hazards, including signs and symptoms of exposure, associated with exposure to chemicals and any medical condition known to be aggravated by exposure to a chemical;
- Procedures to protect against hazards (e.g., personal protective equipment required as well as its proper use and maintenance; work practices or methods to assure proper use and handling of chemicals; and procedures for emergency response);
- Work procedures to follow to assure protection when cleaning hazardous chemical spills and leaks; and

• Where MSDSs are located, how to read and interpret the information on labels and MSDSs and how employees may obtain additional hazard information.

The safety officer or designee will review our employee training program and advise the radiology director on training or retraining needs. Retraining is required when the hazard changes or when a new chemical hazard is introduced into the workplace. But it will also be department policy to provide training regularly in safety meetings to ensure the effectiveness of the program. As part of assessing the training program, the radiology safety officer will obtain input from employees on the training they have received, and their suggestions for improving it.

Contractor Employers

The safety officer, Lois Smith, upon notification by the responsible supervisor, will advise outside contractors in person of any chemical hazards that may be encountered in the normal course of their work on the premises, the labeling system in use, the protective measures to be taken, and the safe handling procedures to be used. In addition, Ms. Smith will notify these individuals of the location and availablility of MSDSs. Each contractor bringing chemicals on-site must provide us with the appropriate hazard information on these substances, including the labels used and the precautionary measures to be taken in working with these chemicals.

Additional Information

All employees, or their designated representatives, can obtain further information on this written program, the hazard communication standard and applicable MSDSs at the office of the safety officer, Room A-5.

Adapted from *Hazard Communication Guidelines for Compliance*, "Sample Hazard Communication Program."*This article on hazardous communication appeared in the Fall, 1992 issue of *Radiology Management*. It is reprinted here with the permission of the author.

LIST OF REFERENCES—VOLUME 1

Abele, J. E. New tools extend value of intravascular therapy. *Diagnostic Imaging.* 12(9):57-63, 1990.

Abrams, H. L. Diagnostic technologies: the increasing role of technology assessment. *Decisions in Imaging Economics.* 3(2):29-34, 1990.

Ackerman, L. Digital storage of images. *Administrative Radiology.* 10(3):43-48, 1991.

Adams, H. G. Technologists staffing at the National Naval Medical Center. *Administrative Radiology.* 10(3):23-27, 1991.

"Advancement Programs in the Workplace." Summit on Manpower. Sudbury, MA. May, 1992, p. 3, 4, 6, 9, 23.

American College of Radiology Committee on Quality Assurance in Mammography, "Mammography Quality Control guidelines."

American College of Radiology, "Medicare Mammography Facility Checklist " Reston VA. March 1993.

American Hospital Publishing and the Linc Group, Inc. Profitable Healthcare Equipment. 1990.

Appleby, C. R. Cool laser won't replace balloon angioplasty. *Health Week.* 4(17):31, 1990.

Appleby, C. R. PET imaging: the elite technology. *Health Week.* 4(17):27-30, 1990.

Appleby, C. R. Running out: a scarcity of radiologic technologists, etc. *Health Week.* January 8, 1990.

Appleby, C. R. Suiting up with PACS. *Health Week.* 4(11): 29-32, 1990.

Aribisala, E.B. Applying the Americans with Disabilities Act to Radiology. *Radiology Management.* 15(2):27, 1993.

Bell, B. Careful strategy necessary for counselling effectively. *South Carolina Business Journal.* December 1987.

Berger, S. and Sudman, S.K. Physician/Hospital Trends for the 1990s Raise Some Red Flags. Healthcare Executive MAR/APRIL, 1992, P. 15.

Berkowitz, D. A. Managing your high-tech future. *Health Care Forum Journal.* 32(5):14-20, 1989.

Bittell, L.R. *What Every Supervisor Should Know.* N.Y.: McGraw Hill Book Company, 1980.

Black, W. C. MSI ferrets out electrical activity, identifies origins. *Diagnostic Imaging.* 13(1):74-76, 1991.

Boehme, J. and Choplin, R. RIS selection criteria part 2. *Administrative Radiology.* 9(10):69-71, 1990.

Bouchard, E. A. A business with a heart. *Continuing Care.* 9(3):22, 1990.

Bouchard, E. A. Consumer relations: another change for human resources. *Radiology Management.* 10(2):32, 1988.

Bouchard, E. A. Focused communication and physician bonding strategies. *Radiology Management.* 11(2):50-51, 1989.

Bowden, A. B. Negotiating a system purchase: 8 principles for protecting your institution's interest. *Health Care Executive.* 7(1):17-19, 1992.

Brice, J. Barriers begin to fall in bone densitometry. *Diagnostic Imaging.* 13(7):63-64, 1991.

Brightbill, T. Disk-contentment? *Health Week.* 4(18):21-25, 1990.

Brink, J. V. IMACS support shift toward enhanced service. *Diagnostic Imaging.* 13(9): 11-16, 1991.

Brotman, J. Breaking down barriers to customer focus. *Entrepreneur.* September 1989:14-16.

Bucci, R. Positron Emission Tomography: Executive Update Administrative Radiology. 12(5):53, 1993.

"Buyers' Guide to Evaluating MR Systems." GE Medical Systems. 1986.

Cannavo, M. J. Fitting PACS technology into the hospital of tomorrow. *Diagnostic Imaging.* 10(11):188-190, 1988.

Cannavo, M. J. Radiology information systems can improve department efficiency. *Diagnostic Radiology.* 10(12):92-95, 1988.

Cannavo, M. J. Small imaging companies capture IMACS market. *Diagnostic Imaging.* 13(9):31-34, 1991.

Cerne, F. Computer tomography alive and well. *Hospitals.* 62(27):65-69, 1988.

Cerne, F. Managing radiology data. *Hospitals.* 62(27):78-81, 1988.

Choplin, R. and Boehme, J. RIS the basics part 1. *Administrative Radiology.* 9(9):35-37, 1990.

"Choosing a Clinical Information System." Hewlett-Packard Company, 1990.

"Clinical Applications of Lasers." Laser Centers of America, 1989.

Coleman, E. PET: clinical positron emission tomography. *Administrative Radiology.* 9(6):34-41, 1990.

Courson, P. "On the Road: Planning and Operating a Mobile Mammography Program." *Administrative Radiology.* 10(4):48-58, 1991.

Cunningham, J. Make your next professional interview a success. *Administrative Radiology.* 9(12):25-28, 1990.

Curran, C. Telling it Like it is: Consultants Speak Out. *Second Source Imaging.* 8(3):52, 1993.

D'Agincourt, L. Lack of reimbursement impedes PET's growth. *Diagnostic Imaging.* 14(2):39-48, 1992.

D'Agincourt, Lori. PET's metabolic potency wins it clinical respect. *Diagnostic Imaging.* 14(1):68-75, 1992.

Davis, D., et al. "Meeting the Challenge—A Multidisciplinary Clinical Ladder Program." *Administrative Radiology.* 10:1 (16-20)91.

DeRosier, D. Using statistics to get the staff you need. *RT Image.* 3(37):1, 4-5, 18-19, 1990.

Dohms, J. *Hazard Communication Guidelines for Compliance,* " Sample Hazard Communication Program." *Radiology Management,* Fall 1992.

Dowd, S. Planning for the radiographer of the future. *Administrative Radiology.* 11(3): 36-43, 1992.

Doyle, E. T. Touring the mind with MSI. *RT Image.* 4(12):1, 4-6, 1991.

Eklund, G. W. and Brenner, R. J. The self-referred patient: a challenge to breast imaging practices. *Administrative Radiology.* 9(11):133-136, 1990.

Ellis, J. Employment Provisions in the ADA Protect Disabled from Discrimination. JMA Notes. Feb. 26, 1993, p. 1.

Eubanks, Paula. Hospitals struggle to respond to the technologist shortage. *Hospitals.* 64(14):32-37, 1990.

Fodor, J. Major equipment purchases: a committee approach. *Health Progress.* 69(10):12-14, 1988.

Friedman, G. Overcoming mammography phobia. *Health Week.* 4(7):19-23, 1990.

Gertman, P. M. Cost-containment measures radiology must respond. *Decisions in Imaging Economics.* 3(2):12-14, 1990.

Good, W. F., et al. PACS in radiology: a perspective. *Decisions in Imaging Economics.* 3(4):27-29, 1990.

Graham, J. Filmless radiology departments: fact or fiction. *Decisions in Technology Economics.* 1(1):11-15, 1988.

Greinacher, C. PACS: the patient care picture goes digital. *Seimens Review.* (4) 1988 pp. 3-7.

Gunther, R. Patient outreach: the key role of mammographic technologists in mammogram compliance. *Administrative Radiology.* 10(3):35-40, 1991.

Hall, L. T. Cardiovascular lasers: a look into the future. *American Journal of Nursing.* 90(7):27-30, 1990.

Hanlon, P. I. and Kaskiw, E. A. Physician bonding: one hospital's experience. *Computers in Healthcare.* 10(3):24-26, 1989.

Hanwell, L. The manpower shortage: it's everybody's problem. *Administrative Radiology.* 11(1):35-41, 1992.

Hatfield, S. PET technology advances into clinical settings. *Advance.* 2(8):1-4, 1989.

Hayden, L. and Nilges, E. Digital radiography with phosphur plates. *Administrative Radiology.* 10(5):44-47, 1991.

Hendee, W. R. Evolution of imaging far from complete. *Diagnostic Imaging.* 13(1):13-21, 1991.

Hendee, W. R. Radiology and physics: prognosis for the future. *Decisions in Imaging Economics.* 1(1):8-12, 1988.

Hendee, W. R. Transforming medical imaging from a craft into a science. *Diagnostic Imaging.* 10(11):97-103, 1988.

Henthorne, B. H. Look up from the book. *Administrative Radiology.* 9(10):47-48, 1990.

Hersey, P. and Blanchard, K. Management of Organizational Behavior. Englewood Cliffs, N.J., Prentice-Hall, Inc. 1982, pp. 41, 42.

Hess, T. P. Complexity of radiology management calls for computerized solutions. *Diagnostic Imaging.* 10(5):69-79, 1988.

Heuerman, J. N. Advice from a Head Hunter. *Healthcare Forum Journal.* 32(4):34-38, 1989.

Hopkins, E. M. A G.R.E.A.T. idea. *Health Progress.* 70(6):82-84, 1989.

Hoppszallern, S. and Handmaker, H. A national PET utilization forecast. *Administrative Radiology.* 11(2):32-37, 1992.

Huang, H. K. Implementing PACS: experience in future plans. *Decisions in Imaging Economics.* 3(2):20-24, 1990.

Hunter, D. P. and Jerew, M. Physician relationships in troubled hospitals. *Hospital Management Review.* 9(10):1, 1990.

Hunter, T. B. The personal computer in the radiologist's office. *Applied Radiology.* 20(8):33-36, 1991.

Institute for Clinical PET. 1991. "Average cost of a clinical PET scan based on procedures at 26 facilities."

Jaffe, C. C. and Lemke, H. U. Computer options open new radiology windows. *Diagnostic Imaging.* 13(9):21-28, 1991.

JCAHO Recommended Plant/Safety Orientation. *New Employee Orientation.*

Johnson, D. Relationship management clearly differentiates hospitals. *Healthcare Strategic Management.* 7(8):2-3, 1989.

Jones, W. J. Letting technology dictate design. *Healthcare Strategic Management.* 6(11):10-12, 1988.

Katzen, B. T. Lasers and other vascular devices may augment balloon angioplasty. *Diagnostic Imaging.* 10(4):55-56, 1988.

Ketchum, L. E. RSNA 1991: technical highlights. *Applied Radiology.* 21(1):62-70, 1992.

King, G. R. Let the employer beware. *Modern Healthcare's Facilities Operation and Management.* 21(18):24-25,1991.

Krug, H. Subsidizing screening mammography through induced revenues and profits. *Radiology Management.* 12(4):28-32, 1990.

Kuber, M. S. Radiologic administration: structure and style. *Radiology Management.* 2(1):6-15, 1980.

Kurzweil Applied Intelligence, Inc. Voice Recognition Generated Report. Walttham, MA.

Langley, M. ADA Expected to change jobs, hiring. The Knoxville News Sentinel, June 27, 1993.

Lester, B. *Verifying references.* Johnstown, PA.

Lester, B. *What You Can and Can't Ask During an Interview.* Johnstown, PA.

Levine, B. and Bozarth, C. A guide to PACS-RIS/HIS communication. *Administrative Radiology.* 11(1):43-47, 1992.

Linn, B. Hospital use lags behind laser's tremendous potential. *Healthcare Strategic Management.* 7(8):1, 19-23, 1989.

Lumsdon, K. Moving target: hospitals take careful steps in acquiring PET. *Hospitals.* 66(7):58-62, 1992.

Lynch, Maureen. Department directors provide the steps to heavenly imaging. *Administrative Radiology.* 11(3):51-53, 1992.

Mace, J. Approaching clinical advancement in radiology. *Radiology Management.* 13(4):45, 1991.

"Magnetic Resonance Imagers." *Healthweek.* November, 1990.

Maner, P. and Hamilton, T. The team approach. *Administrative Radiology.* 11(2):39-43, 1992.

"Manpower Networking Resource." *Summit on Manpower.* 1990.

Mayer, J. Find the Job You've Always Wanted in Half the Time and with Half the Effort (1992) Contemporary Books. Adapted by *The Pryor Report* Vol 9(1):9, 1993.

McCue, P. The shortage of radiologic technologists. *Applied Radiology.* 19(5):28-31, 1989.

Melbin, J. E. Challenging the gold standard. *RT Image.* 5(3):4-9, 1992.

Melbin, J. E. Hyperthermia: the fourth frontier. *RT Image.* 9(29):1, 4-6, 35, 1991.

Meyer, P., et al. The American College of Radiology Mammography Accreditation Program. *Administrative Radiology.* 9(8):28-36, 1990.

Mitigui, J. The waiting room. *Health Progress.* 68(1):122, 1987.

Nabi, H. A. Antibody imaging in colon cancer. *Applied Radiology.* 21(2):59-64, 1992.

Nelson, M. The shortage of radiologic technologists. *Decisions in Imaging Economics.* 2(1):20-25, 1990.

News Briefs: Bush signs mammography bill. *Second Source Imaging.* 8(1):14,1993.

New Britain MRI. Sample floor plan of MRI facility. New Britain, Conn.

Nielsen, G. A. How to make salary comparisons and negotiate a raise. *Radiology Management.* 13(1):52-3, 1991.

Nowak, S. Patient power: a commentary. *Administrative Radiology.* 11(2):55, 1992.

O'Leary, T. J., et al. Screening mammography: barriers and incentives. *Applied Radiology.* 20(9):11-17, 1991.

"PACS: A NEMA Primer." The National Electrical Manufacturers Association, 1988.

"PACS Components." *Healthweek.* June 11, 1990.

"PACS in Place in the United States." *Diagnostic Imaging*: Focus on PACS. September, 1990.

Parker, M. A. Risk of malpractice escalates in breast cancer screening. *Diagnostic Imaging.* 10(7):82-85, 1988.

Peterson, K. Caring for people, not profits, brings success. *Modern Healthcare.* 20(39):34, 1990.

Powills, S. Mobile technology takes radiology on the road. *Hospitals.* 62(21):80,1988.

Press, I. and Gainey, R. What experiences contribute to satisfaction with the hospital? *Michigan Hospitals.* September 1990, pp. 17-21.

Rooney, M. Resume rules for healthcare executives. *Healthcare Executive.* 6(4):35, 1991.

Rowe, W. M. Upgrading a radiology information system. *Radiology Management.* 12(2):24-28, 1990.

Rowe, W. Purchase considerations for a radiology information system. *Radiology Management.* 14(1):43-45, 1992.

Ryan, K. and Oestreich, D. *Driving Fear Out of the Workplace*, Jossey-Bass: San Francisco, CA. Adapted by *The Pryor Report*, Vol 19(1):8, 1993.

Schmitz, S., et al. The current status of bone densitometry. *Applied Radiology.* 19(6):20-26, 1990.

Schwartz, H. W. Evaluating productivity and budgeting staff. *Radiology Management.* 11(3):39, 1989.

Schwartz, H. W. Practical considerations in evaluating a radiology information management system for your environment. *Radiology Management.* 13(3):30-35, 1991.

Schwartz, H.W. "Justifying Capital Equipment in the 1990's." *Radiology Management.* 12(2):35-39, 1990.

Seago, K. Scoring a radiology department's niceness factor. *Applied Radiology*. 15(1):49-51, 1986.

Seshadri, S. B. Mini-PACS help solve image problems today. *Diagnostic Imaging*. 13(9):17-19, 1991.

Siemens/CTI PET Systems Nuclear PET Group. Knoxville, TN.

Skillington, C.J. "Directory of Technologist Education in MRI." *R.T. Image Magazine*. Oct. 26, 1992.

Skjei, E. UCLA tackles obstacles to filmless department. *Diagnostic Imaging*. 13(9):3-9, 1991.

Solomon, A. and Martino, S. Relative value units: practical productivity management. *Radiology Management*. 13(1):33-35, 1991.

Southwick, K. MABS: the imaging phenom. *Health Week*. 4(22):62-64, 1990.

Stockburger, W. T. and King, W. E. PACS: a financial analysis for economic viability. *Applied Radiology*. 19(1):17-24, 1990.

Straub, W. H. and Dey, A. A. So you want to get into the breast imaging business? *Administrative Radiology*. 8(7):14-17, 1989.

"Summit on Manpower, Report: April 1989." Summit on Manpower.

"Tech shortage spurs Summit actions." *ACR Bulletin*. vol. 47(3), 1991.

"Technology on Wheels: Evaluating the Options." *Health Technology*. 1(6):231-238, 1987.

Tighe, L.C. PET: When Will it Get Here? *Second Source Imaging*. 7(12):40-2, 1992.

Tilke, B. Equipment purchases demand skill savvy—and specifics. *Advance*. 3(35): 1-9, 1990.

Tsuchiyama, S. Difficult questions: treating the self-referred patient. *Administrative Radiology*. 9(11):129-132, 1990.

Wachel, W. Do you know your physicians? *Healthcare Executive*. 7(2):14-17, 1992.

Wagner, M. "Keep Unique...for PET" *Modern Healthcare*. November 30, 1992.

Wagner, M. Establishing Pet Charges Requires Identification of Total Costs. *Modern Healthcare*. November 30, 1992. p. 38.

Wagner, M. Weighing the costs of new technology. *Modern Healthcare*. 18(34):43-58, 1988.

Walklett, W. and Green, J. Heat as a diagnostic aid. *Administrative Radiology*. 9(12):57-59, 1990.

Walt, A. J. Screening and breast cancer: a surgical perspective. *American College of Surgeons Bulletin*. 75(9):6-10, 1990.

Wedel, C.S. The Americans with Disabilities Act: The Impact on Radiologic Technologists and Managers. *Radiology Management*, 15(2):23, 1993.

Weinstein, A. Hospitals should say no to some technologies. *Hospitals.* 64(18):80, 1990.

Weiss, R. Appealing to an important customer. *Health Progress.* 70(4):38-45, 1989.

Wesolowski, C. E. Show that you care. *Radiology Management.* 12(4):34-38, 1990.

West, Michael G. Information system can save money while improving patient care. *Diagnostic Imaging.* 10(5):159-162, 1988.

Whelan, M.C. Getting to the Bone. *Second Source Imaging.* 7(4): 50-57, 1992.

Wood, C. J. How much does an employee really cost? *RT Image.* 3(43):1, 6, 7, 21, 1990.

Worth, J. Your crystal image: developing your resume. *Administrative Radiology.* 9(12):22-24, 1990.

LIST OF REFERENCES—VOLUME 2

"Administrator's Guide to MR." GE Medical Systems, 1990.

"A Layman's Guide to Hospitals: An Introduction to Finance and Economics." Coopers and Lybrand, 1978.

Albrecht, K. *Service Within*, Dow Jones-Irwin, Homewood, IL. As adapted by The Pryor Report Vol 9(1):9, 1993.

Anderson, H. J. Survey identifies trends in equipment acquisitions. *Hospitals.* 64(18):30, 32-35, 1990.

Annis, R . Budgeting: getting to the bottom line. *Health Progress.* December 1988, pp. 74-76.

Annis, R. Accounts receivable: how to monitor and control them. *Health Progress.* May 1988, pp. 70-71.

Appleby, C. R. Spreading the word: hospitals market imaging services by educating consumers, physicians. *Health Week.* 4(5):37-43, 1990.

Arbeiter, J. S. Are you merely a witness to the patient's consent? *RN* 51(10):53-57, 1988.

ARC Standard for Communication—Diagnostic Radiology. *ACR Bulletin.* 11/91.

Bartlett, E. E. Talk to your patients to avoid trouble later with malpractice. *Diagnostic Imaging.* 9(11):179-187, 1987.

Bergey, T. W. Sorting out the three r's: RVU, RVS and RBRVS. *Radiology Management.* 13(4):35-39, 1991.

Bogardus, C. Billing tactics: advantages of a professional billing service in radiation oncology. *Administrative Radiology.* 10(1):51-56, 1991.

Bonnis, N., Micheletti, J., and Shlala, T. CQI Initiatives: Impact on Radiology. *Administrative Radiology.* 12(10):24. 1992.

Bouchard, E. Service line management. *Radiology Management.* 14(1):22-23, 1992.

Bradley, L. Industry strategies have appropriate home in hospitals. *Healthcare Strategic Management.* 8(6):8-13, 1990.

Brice, J. "Simple Tactics Minimize Exposure to Malpractice." *Diagnostic Imaging.* 14(3):44-45, 1992.

Brice, J. CON regs loosen grip on imaging equipment. *Diagnostic Imaging.* 12(9):73-76, 1990.

Brown, S. W. and Morley, A. P. Marketing through the medical staff. *Healthcare Executive.* 1(2):45-48, 1986.

Brown, S.W. and Morley, A.P. *Marketing Strategies for Physicians.* Oradell, NJ, Medical Economics Books. 1986, p. 130.

Brumbaugh, J., et al. Conversion to nonionics packs economic punch. *Diagnostic Imaging.* 13(7):99-104, 1991.

Buff, H. "Preparing for the JCAH survey." *Administrative Radiology.* 6(7):28-32, 1987.

Burke, M. Chilling effect on mergers? *Trustee.* 43(8):20-21, 1990.

"Buyers Guide to Evaluating MR Systems." GE Medical Systems, 1986.

Byers, K. D. and Livingston, C. A framework for writing a business plan. Management Issues. Peat Marwick Main and Company, 1989.

Carswell, H. Older MRI systems yield $500,000± in profits. *Diagnostic Imaging.* 13(7):41-44, 1991.

Chapman-Cliburn, G. Risk management and quality assurance: issues and interactions. *Quality Review Bulletin.* 1986.

"Coaching and Counselling." Stewart and Associates, Inc., Columbia, SC, 1990.

Conley, D. J. and Greenberg, J. Financial considerations in purchasing technical equipment. *The Journal of Medical Practice Management.* 3(1):23-26, 1987.

"Creating a Winning Marketing Campaign." American Management Association, 1990.

Curran, C. Government regulations. *Second Source Imaging.* 7(3):32-38, 1992.

Dey, A. The ABC's of billing. *Administrative Radiology.* 9(4):39-41, 1990.

Di Giacinto, T. M., et al. The MRI decision process. *Administrative Radiology.* 9(1):27-30, 1990.

Dickes, L. *Reimbursement Lingo* from "Influencing Reimbursement." *RT Image.* 3(27): 16-17, 1990.

DiStefano, M. and Orlandi, A. V. Historical facts regarding limited licensure. *RT Image.* 3(40):5, 22, 1990.

Dowd, S. Planning for the radiographer of the future. *Administrative Radiology.* 11(3):36-43, 1992.

Doyle, E. T. The fight for licensure goes on. *RT Image.* 4(31):10-11, 36-37, 1991.

Drane, J. F. and Roth, R. B. Medical decision making for the incompetent patient. *Health Progress.* 68(12):37-42, 1987.

Drew, P. G. Walking the tightrope bridging cost and quality. *Diagnostic Imaging.* 13(7):57-60, 1991.

"Eleven Safe Harbors to Find." *ACR Bulletin.* 47(9):1, 4-11, 1991.

Eubanks, P. Acclamating the new exec should be first goal. *Hospitals.* 65(5):50, 1991.

Eubanks, P. Clinicians: manage your move to manager. *Hospitals.* 65(5):60, 1991.

Examples of Monitoring and Evaluation in Diagnostic Radiology, Radiation Oncology and Nuclear Medicine Services. Chicago: JCAHO, 1988.

Faden, A. I. and Faden, R. R. Informed consent in medical practice: with particular reference to neurology. *Archives of Neurology.* 35(11):761-764, 1978.

Fischer, H. W. Raising department efficiency with concentric zone design. *Diagnostic Imaging.* 10(9):168-170, 1988.

Fisk, T. A. The marketing matrix: adopting an analytic approach. *Decisions in Imaging Economics.* 2(4):12-19, 1989.

Gardner, E. UB-82 forms offer wealth of information, misinformation. *Modern Healthcare.* 20(38):18-29,1990.

Glossary of JCAHO Terms. *JCAHO Accreditation Manual for Hospitals.* 1992.

Goldsmith, M. and Leebov, W. Strengthening the hospital's marketing position through training. *Healthcare Management Review.* 11(2):83-93, 1986.

Green, A. M. RVS puts radiologists at forefront in medicine's search for values. *Diagnostic Imaging.* 11(6):63-66, 1989.

Greene, J. "A Strategy for Cutting Back: screening processes mark money–losing services for closing. *Modern Healthcare.* 19(33):29-47, 1989.

Gur, D., et al. A perspective of the resource-based relative value scale. *Administrative Radiology.* 10(3):28-34, 1991.

Hansen, R. F. Increasing market share through good design. *Healthcare Strategic Management.* 5(3):15-21, 1987.

Harms, S. Magnetic resonance imaging. *Administrative Radiology.* 9(8):39-49,1990.

Hatfield, S. Administrators look to build confidence in construction decisions. *Advance.* 4(32):24-25, 1991.

Hatfield, S. RT's and the law: a few precautions can reduce risk of lawsuits. *Advance.* 2(10):14-15, 1989.

Hayward, J. 1992 CPT coding changes. *Administrative Radiology.* 11(3):45-47, 1992.

Healthweek—Desktop Resource. Healthcare Knowledge Systems (CPHA). September 24, 1990. Ann Arbor, MI.

Hess, T. P. Personal contact, not a hard sell, wins referrals for MRI services. *Diagnostic Imaging.* 10(3):67-72, 1988.

"History of the ARRT Involvement with State Licensure." ARRT Annual Report, 1989. p. 3.

Hoppszallern, S. MRI: a forecast for the future. *Administrative Radiology.* 9(8):51-55, 1990.

"How safe are your harbors?" *Imaging Economics.* Vol. 1, No. 1, March 1992. p. 7.

"How Should Stereotactic Breast Biopsy be Coded?" The RMBA Bulletin. November 1992. Costa Mesa, CA.

"How to Use CPT Coding." Medi-Index Publications. Salt Lake City, Utah. 6(3):3, 1991.

Hudson, T. Hospital/MD joint ventures move forward despite hurdles. *Hospitals.* 65(9):22-28, 1991.

Hughes, C. and Van Gilse, M. Tracking the elusive MRI referral pattern. *Administrative Radiology.* 9(11):111-114, 1990.

Hughes, C. Consider financial options prior to leasing equipment. *Diagnostic Imaging.* 11(8):40-41, 137, 1989.

Hughes, C.M. "MRI centers must sell themselves to survive in competitive market." *Diagnostic Imaging.* 10(7):95, 1988.

Hulley SB, Cummings SR, eds. *Designing Clinical Research: An Epidemiologic Approach.* Baltimore: Williams & Wilkins, 1988, p.43. Imaging Economics Newsletter. Vol, No. 4, 1993, p. 2.

Hunton, B. W. Good planning takes organization. *Advance.* 4(32):24-25, 1991.

Hunton, B.W. Protocols: Guide use of non-ionic contrast media. Advance for Administrators. 2(5):11, 1992.

Iglehart, J. K. and White, J. K. Hospital industry divided on Medicare capital payments. *Health Progress.* 68(1):17-18, 93, 1987.

"Improving Report Turnaround Time to Increase Referrals." *Imaging Market Forum.* 5(2):1-5, 1988.

"IRS Acts on Joint Ventures." *ACR Bulletin.* 48(2):1, 5-6, 1992.

Jablonski, J.R. Implementing Total Quality Management in the 1990's. Technical Management Consortium, Inc. Albuquerque, N.M., 1991, p. 81.

Johnson, G. Total quality management: will it work for me? *Radiology Management.* 14(1):30-31, 1992.

Johnson, K. C. MRI centers: ten design mistakes to avoid. *Hospitals.* 61(7):82-84, 1987.

Jones-Bey, H. Radiologists in quandary over ethics of nonionics. *Diagnostic Imaging.* 14(2):9-15, 1992.

Kanal, E. Taking a logical approach to MRI system acquisition. *Diagnostic Imaging.* 10(8):73-80, 182, 1988.

Katayama, H. The contrast media controversy: implications of a landmark safety study. *Administrative Radiology.* 9(9):20-22, 1990.

Keefe, J. and Sullivan, R. New planning assumptions needed in deregulated imaging climate. *Diagnostic Imaging.* 9(10):71-75, 1987.

Keenan, L. A. and Goldman, E. F. "Positive Imaging: Design as Marketing Tool in Diagnostic Centers." *Administrative Radiology.* 8(2):36-41, 1989.

Keenan, L. Design and architecture in radiology. *Administrative Radiology.* 9(6):43-48, 1990.

Kidd, K. L. Radiology reimbursement. *Applied Radiology.* 18(5):16-21, 1989.

Koska, M.T., JCAHO Introduces three new areas of survey concentration. *Hospitals.* Oct. 5, 1992, pp. 62-64.

Kropf, R. Developing a competitive advantage in the market for radiology services. *Hospital and Health Services Administration.* 33(2):213-220, 1988.

Kukla, S. F. *Cost Accounting and Financial Analysis for the Hospital Administrator.* American Hospital Publishing, Inc., 1986.

Kuntz, L. A. Medical negligence. *RT Image.* 5(1):4-5, 17, 1992.

Kyes, K. A Nationwide Review. *Decisions in Imaging Economics.* Vol. 5, No. 3, 1992.

Labovitz, G. H. Beyond the total quality management mystique. *Healthcare Executive.* 6(2):15-17, 1991.

Lawson, T. C. Joint ventures: a legal evaluation. *Decisions in Imaging Economics.* 3(3): 1990.

Leckie, R. et al. Surveying for Excellence in Radiology. *Administrative Radiology.* 12(8):34, 1992.

Leiter, P. and Jacobson, S. L. "Sound Marketing for Off Site Private Practices." *Rehab Management.* 4(6):37-40, 1990.

Lille, K. "Applying for a Certificate of Need." *Radiology/Nuclear Medicine Magazine.* 7(4):29, 1977.

Long, H. W. Cash flow, capital costs and provider incentives. *Decisions in Imaging Economics.* 3(4):22-26, 1990.

"Low Osmolality Contrast Media: Choice and Challenge for the '80's." Special Supplement. *Diagnostic Imaging.* 9(12):1-32, 1987.

Lucchese, D. R. and Eikman, E. A. The medical-legal implications of contrast agent use. *Applied Radiology.* 18(12):36-37, 1989.

Lynch, Maureen. Department directors provide the steps to heavenly imaging. *Administrative Radiology.* 11(3):51-53, 1992.

Lynch, R. "Reimbursement Management Primer for DRG and ICD-9 Analysis." *Journal of Cardiovascular Management.* 2(1):41-48, 1990.

"Magnetic Resonance Glossary." Siemens Medical Systems, Inc., 1988.

Maltzer, R. The hazards of outcome measures. *Administrative Radiology.* 11(1):51-52, 1992.

Maner, P. and Hamilton, T. The team approach. *Administrative Radiology.* 11(2):39-43, 1992.

"Market-based strategies boost imaging referrals." *Diagnostic Imaging.* 15(1):23, 1993.

"Marketing: A Four Step Process." *The Medical Network: Emergency and Convenience Care News.* September 1988, pp. 3-4.

Martin, J. Maslow and manpower: a humanistic approach to technologist retention. *RT Image.* 2(31):10-12, 1989.

Matson, Holleman, Nosek and Wilkinson. *The Journal of Family Practice.* 36(2): 204-205, 1993.

McAtte, J. A. Practical guidelines to responding to court subpeonas. _The Journal of Medical Practice Management._ 3(1):47-51, 1987.

McCue, P. "Consultant Services in Quality Assurance and Risk Management." _Applied Radiology._ 17(11):23-24, 1988.

McCue, P. Diagnostic imaging centers: turnkeys complete. _Applied Radiology._ 16(9): 27-34, 1987.

McIlrath, S. Bad news on RBRVS rules. _AMA News._ June 17, 1991, pp. 1, 28-29.

Meehan, C.H. "The Guide to Department Planning." Columbia, S.C.

Mescon, M. H. and Mescon, T. S. Leading by inspiration: an example. _Sky._ 20(4):102-104, 1991.

Mescon, M. H. and Mescon, T. S. One customer at a time. _Sky._ 20(2):100-101, 1991.

Miccio, J. A. The migration of medical technology. _Healthcare Forum Journal._ 32(5):23-26, 1989.

Michael, K. The evolution of continuing education in the field of allied health. _Administrative Radiology._ 11(1):27-28, 1992.

Morrison, J. Malpractice issues in the education of healthcare professionals, part 1. _Advance._ 2(14):1-3, 28, 1989.

Morrison, J. Malpractice issues in the education of healthcare professionals, part 2. _Advance._ 2(15):7-9, 1989.

Motyka, E. A step above: marketing the cancer center. _Administrative Radiology._ 9(9):51-52, 1990.

Musfeldt, C. The Last Word: 10 Attributes of a hassle-free hospital. _Hospitals._ August 20, 1992. p. 76.

Newbold, P. A. Emerging new relationships: from the customer's perspective. _Hospital Entrepreneur's Newsletter._ 3(1):4-7, 1987.

"Nonionic Contrast Media: Selective or 100% Usage?" Special Supplement. _Diagnostic Imaging._ 89(12):1-20, 1990.

Nowak, S. F. Living with the budget. _Applied Radiology._ 17(10):28, 77-78, 1989.

Nyberg, M. Turn around time: a financially troubled Philadelphia hospital goes out of the red and into the black. _Health Progress._ 72(7):57-61, 1991.

O'Dell, C. Building on received wisdom. _Healthcare Forum Journal._ 36(1): 17-8, 1993.

Olsen, G. G. Business venture restrictions. _Rehab Management._ 5(1):106-107, 1992.

"Organization Directory: 1992." _Administrative Radiology._ 11(1):55-61, 1992.

"Organizations in Radiology." American College of Radiology, 1990.

"Patient Satisfaction Survey." American Healthcare Radiology Administrators, 1993.

Placone, R. C. and Farr, M. H. Steering a center from startup to success. *Administrative Radiology*. 9(2):36-40, 1990.

Placone, R. C. The mid-field MRI center: 1990's answer to the continuing crisis in healthcare costs. *Administrative Radiology*. 9(10):55-62, 1990.

"Planning a new MRI Facility: Avoiding Common Mistakes." *Imaging Economics*. Vol. 1, No. 3, 1992.

"Potential Antitrust Violations." *ACR Bulletin*. 47(6):16-18, 1991.

"Preparing a Business Plan: A Guide for the Emerging Company." Ernst and Whinney, 1987.

Primer on Indicator Development and Application: Measuring Quality in Health Care. JCAHO, 1990.

"Principles for a Sound Quality Effort." *The Westrend Letter*. September 1990, p. 3.

"Professional Organizations." *1992 Radiology Reference Guide*. Access Publishing Co., pp. 161-164.

"Radiology Reimbursement Reference: To Guide You Through the Maze of Radiology Reimbursement." American Healthcare Radiology Administrators, 1990.

Reuter, S. R. An overview of informed consent for radiologists. *AJR*. 148:219-227, 1987.

Rollo, F. D. Patient protection: utilizing quality control measures for success. *Decisions in Imaging Economics*. 3(5):4-7, 1990.

Roper, R. R. How to loose informed consent. *Applied Radiology*. 18(4):8-10, 1989.

Rostenberg, B., Campbell, J., and Stein, M. "Managing Successful Radiology Projects." RSNA '92 presentation. Chicago, Ill.

Rudnick, J. D. A process and considerations for activating a quality/productivity monitoring system. *Healthcare Strategic Management*. 5(3):23-27, 1987.

Sackett, M. H. "Quality Assurance Management: the Reasons and Results." *Radiology Management*. 11(2)1989:54-55.

Schonfeld, A. R. Marketing radiology to referring physicians. *Applied Radiology*. 17(11):9, 1988.

Schonfeld, A. R. Teleradiology: examining its impact on imaging management. *Decisions in Imaging Economics*. 2(4):20-25, 1989.

Schwartz, H. W. Justifying capital equipment in the 1990's. *Radiology Management*. 12(2):35-39, 1990.

Schwartz, H. W. Managing radiology in the 1990's, part 1. *Applied Radiology*. 19(7):13-16, 1990.

Scott, C. and Jaffe, T. *Managing Organizational Change*, Crisp Publications. Los Altos, CA. As adapted by the Pryor Report Vol 9(1):6, 1993.

Seago, K. Imaging center design and construction: good planning pays off. *Applied Radiology.* 16(2):37-42, 1987.

Seaver, D. J. Taking charge: winning strategies for hospital CEOs in new positions. *Healthcare Executive.* 5(6):13-16, 1990.

"Self-referral Deplored." *ACR Bulletin.* 48(1):1, 4-5, 1992.

Shorr, A. S. Structuring and negotiating the deal. *Healthcare Strategic Management.* 5(8):4-7, 1987.

Simmons, J. E. Holding marketing accountable. *California Hospitals.* 2(4):18-21, 1988.

"Six Steps to Choosing the Right Corporate Consultant." *Hospitals.* 65(13):45, 1991.

Smith, P. A. Uncover the hidden technical component. *Update.* 6(3):1-5, 1991.

Solomon, M. A. Put emotions aside when assessing whether or not to open MRI center. *Diagnostic Imaging.* 10(11):163-169, 1988.

"Sound Planning and Design for Technology-Related Construction: The Ultimate High Technology." *Health Technology.* 1(6):247-254, 1987.

Spring, D. B. Radiologists approach concensus on informed consent procedures. *Diagnostic Imaging.* 10(11):171-172, 1988.

"Staff Gains Confidence in Total Quality Management Through Its Use in Effective Problem-Solving at 500-bed Medical Center Hospital of Vermont." *Healthcare Productivity Report.* 4(2):1-7, 1991.

"Starting and Managing Your Radiology Imaging Center." *Winthrop Pharmaceuticals—Diagnostic Imaging Division.*

Steel, J. and Perry, J. Reducing repeat films through a total quality Management Approach. *Administrative Radiology.* 11(2):47-49, 1992.

Stewart, D. Equipment leasing: a guide for lessees. *Administrative Radiology.* 9(2):87-90, 1990.

Stier, R. D. Creating an effective marketing team. *Healthcare Executive.* 4(3):36-38, 1987.

Stone, D. A. How to prepare a radiology policy and procedure manual. *Radiology Management.* 2(2):16-20, 1980.

"Strategic Planning Doesn't Stop With the Plan." *Optimal Health.* 3(4):25, 1987.

Straub, W. and Gur, D. Optimizing performance of the billing company. *Administrative Radiology.* 10(1):38-40, 1991.

Studnicki, J. Measuring service line competitive position: a systematic methodology for hospitals. *Health Progress.* 72(6):68-72, 1991.

Templeton, N. Procedural coding evolves. *ACR Bulletin.* 48(1):9-11, 1992.

Tilke, B. RT's continue to wage battle for licensure. *Advance.* 3(43):1-2, 9, 1988.

Tokarski, C. Revised Stark bill still packs enough wallop to slow ventures. *Modern Healthcare.* 19(29):34-36, 1989.

"Top 25 Most Frequently Performed Radiology Procedures." Healthcare Knowledge Systems (CPHA). Ann Arbor, MI. *Healthweek—Desktop Resource. September 24, 1990.*

Trout, M. E. and Bernard, J. A. "Integrity is the Real Bottom Line." *Trustee.* 41(12):11, 1988.

Tsuchiyama, S. How to build the perfect technologist. *Administrative Radiology.* 9(12):44-52, 1990.

Urban, C. D. Market-driven communication strategy. *The Healthcare Forum Journal.* 34(1):24-27, 50, 1991.

Wagner, M. Promoting hospital's high-tech equipment. *Modern Healthcare.* 18(47):43-48, 62-58, 1988.

Wagner, S. K. IRS policy raises another barrier to joint venturing. *Diagnostic Imaging.* 14(2):24, 1992.

Walters, N. R. Conducting special events in malls. *Public Relations Journal.* November 1989, pp. 31-33.

Weatherington, R. Avoiding wrongful discharge suits. *Cardiology Management.* 1(3):14-21, 1987.

Weber, D. Alta Bates-Herrick Hospital implements service line management model, dismantles traditional nursing department. *Healthcare Organization Report.* 1(1):1-12, 1988.

Weinstein, A. Radiology Benchmarking. *Decisions in Imaging Economics.* Winter 1992.

Wilbanks, J. and Mori, K. "Quality Management: Radiology's Challenge." *Administrative Radiology.* 9(10):50-54, 1990.

Wilson, C. N. and Benn, S. A. The medicare catastrophic coverage act of 88: effects on radiology services. *Applied Radiology.* 18(3):19-22, 1989.

Wolff, G. Nonionic agents: okay they're safer—now what? *Administrative Radiology.* 9(11):92-106, 1990.

"Working with Consultants." *Healthcare Dynamics.* 1(6):1990.

Wortley, D. W. and Payne, G. R. Understanding the medicare cost report. *Health Administration Today.* 1(1):23-27, 1988.

Wright, M.L. "Communicating Through Codes." *AHRA Radiology Reimbursement Reference: To Guide You Through the Maze of Radiology Reimbursement.* AHRA. Sudbury, MA, 1991.

Zampetti, J. Predesign facilities for change. *Healthcare Strategic Management.* 8(4):12-14, 1990.

Zampetti, J. The plan to expand. *Administrative Radiology.* 9(10):65-67, 1990.

Zelch, J. V. Educated referral based leads to successful MRI practice. *MRI Quarterly.* Fall 1991.

INDEX—VOLUME 1

INDEX—VOLUME 2